THE ... ...

The brains behind the beauty of some of India's biggest celebrities, Yasmin Karachiwala is also widely credited with bringing Pilates to India. Her list of certifications include BASI (Body Arts and Science International) Certified Pilates Instructor, Balanced Body Comprehensive Master Instructor, Balanced Body MOTR Master Instructor, Balanced Body Bodhi Master Instructor, Balanced Body Core Align Master Instructor, Balanced Body Barre Instructor, ACE (American Council of Exercise) Certified Personal Instructor, Fletcher Pilates Instructor, Core Suspend Instructor, Core Barre Instructor, Core Reform Instructor, Certified Cardiolates Instructor, Certified Konnector Instructor, among others. Her multidisciplinary approach to fitness includes weight training, HIIT, cardio, functional training, Pilates and more, and can be accessed at the Yasmin Karachiwala Body Image (YKBI) chain of studios located both in India and internationally.

Her clients past and present include Katrina Kaif, Alia Bhatt, Deepika Padukone, Kareena Kapoor Khan, Sophie Choudry, Hrithik Roshan, Kiara Advani, Malaika Arora, Karisma Kapoor, Amrita Arora, Neha Dhupia, Arjun Rampal, Kunal Kapoor, Ajit Agarkar, Zaheer Khan, Hardik Pandya, Kriti Sanon, Vaani Kapoor, Bipasha Basu, Preity Zinta, Huma Qureshi, Sonakshi Sinha, Ananya Panday and Sonam Kapoor Ahuja. Hugely popular on Instagram, she can be followed @yasminkarachiwala.

She lives with her family in Mumbai. And with her dog Enzo, who is the biggest celebrity of them all.

This is her first solo book.

Celebrating 35 Years of
Penguin Random House India

ADVANCE PRAISE FOR YASMIN AND *THE PERFECT 10:*
*10-MINUTE WORKOUTS YOU CAN DO ANYWHERE*

'In this fast-paced world that we live in, we often neglect our physical, mental and emotional well-being. I've always believed in the power of nurturing my mind and body consistently, even if it is for just 10 minutes a day, making *The Perfect 10: 10-Minute Workouts You Can Do Anywhere* my perfect companion'—**Deepika Padukone**, actor

'Workouts with Yas are always a surprise—it's never the same and it's always evolving! One of the things I look for when I exercise is to truly cut off from the rest of the world, visiting that safe place that leaves you feeling alive and rejuvenated after—and that's exactly how I feel after a Pilates session with Yas! Whether it's after a super long night shoot or before a big song sequence or right in the middle of my third trimester of pregnancy, the way she constructs workouts is fully tailored to my needs at that moment and that's why the 60 minutes I spend working out with Yas leaves me feeling *beyond* great! This book will leave *you* feeling the same way; I can give it to you in writing! :)'—**Alia Bhatt**, actor

'It is really inspiring to see Yasmin when she is in her element at the gym because she is so passionate and knowledgeable about her craft. The thing I admire most about Yasmin, which is also one of the reasons that has kept us training together for so long, is that she is constantly improving herself and her skills and learning something new. I think the 10-minute workout stacks are great. You have to keep moving every day and that's really important'—**Katrina Kaif**, actor

'Yasmin is one hell of an instructor! She is the best in the business! When I am in a session with her, there is no frivolous talk, no pandering; just pure energy and a laser focus on technique and form, which she exudes with a kindness that is essential. Pilates can make you feel vulnerable no matter how strong you are, and she makes you feel safe. Her passion for what she does is contagious, and the fact that she continues to grow and learn is something I really admire. I know what her workouts have done for me, and it's amazing! Her workouts target so many areas that most others don't. In my interviews, whenever I speak about fitness, I repeatedly say that you do not need to spend one hour or 45 minutes in the gym for it to be counted as a workout. I am a huge believer in spending even 10–15 minutes a day, time that all of us can extract! So there really are no excuses! I am extremely happy that someone like Yasmin has come out with a 10-minute plan, which I think will empower many people to work out. You only have one life and one body to call your own! At least once in your life, you must give your body a chance to be the best it can be. Starting off with 10 minutes a day can do the trick if you're just consistent. And who better to do it with than the best in the business: Yasmin'—**Hrithik Roshan**, actor

'I've known Yasmin for thirty years, and the first place we trained together was my home gym at Galaxy. Yasmin was the first one to get Pilates to India, and a lot of people have and continue to benefit from it. She has also brought the first Pilates festival to the country. If I have to train in Pilates, then I would train with nobody else but Yasmin'—**Salman Khan**, actor

'For me, Pilates (and Yas) entered my life at a time I needed it the most. I was recovering from an injury and needed to strengthen small muscles that made a big difference to my game. Yas was a big help and looked after me well beyond her professional capacity. Pilates helped me work on muscles that a lot of gym exercises do not cover and improved my mobility greatly. Before I started these sessions, I always thought Pilates was for women, but when I did it, I realized that everyone could benefit from it. I think Pilates is a game-changer and Yas is the best'—**Hardik Pandya**, cricketer

'Yasmin is the queen of fitness! Her 10-minute routine is magical and the answer to not just me but to so many millions who don't have the time to work out. This book is pure gold'—**Karan Johar**, filmmaker

'I began my fitness journey with Yasmin way before my film debut. She gave me my foundation in fitness—a holistic approach to a healthier lifestyle. What I love about her the most is her passion for learning and growing. For as long as I've known her, I've seen her travel the world to ensure that she stays updated with the best of the best in the field of fitness'—**Kiara Advani**, actor

'Yasmin was the first one to introduce me to fitness before I even started working out at YKBI (Yasmin Karachiwala's Body Image)—

back to when I was about five years old, and I would watch my mom train with her. Growing up, I always saw her mix fitness with fun, encourage listening to the body and blend flexibility with strength. The idea of a "workout for 10 minutes a day" is something I believe in strongly and try to follow myself because getting in some sort of movement every day is the boost your body needs, and the flexibility of the programmes is what makes it so special. I can't wait to mix it up and try all the workouts'—**Ananya Panday**, actor

'I started training with her for a specific role in a film and she helped me attain a certain fitness level. Ever since then, I have just loved working out with her. Contrary to perception, someone like me needs constant motivation for my workouts and Yasmin has instilled in me a level of discipline and consistency for them and ensured that I do not give in to my comfort zone. On a personal note, Yas is a very genuine friend, and she brings out the best in people; she is caring, warm and amazingly positive'—**Vaani Kapoor**, actor

'I have seen Yas, especially during COVID times, train friends of mine in very innovative ways using whatever time and space that was accessible at that time. This is the perfect time for a book like this to come out, which is about fitness that is accessible to everyone. This book also reminds us that it doesn't need to be complicated or time-consuming but that a little bit is always better than nothing and is a good place to start'—**Vicky Kaushal**, actor

'I started working out with Yasmin to regain my strength after a neck slipped disc but in the process, she and my trainer Prashant at YKBI helped me find a deep love for Pilates. After working out with Yasmin, my body is incredibly different, and I am fitter now than I was in my twenties! I have done her 10-minute stacks and I can say they're amazing. I think this concept could help anyone who feels they don't have time and these workouts also target different body parts; they're fun! So even if I am on the go, and I can't get the time, I will make it a point to add these to my routine. All that *gyaan* about not needing too much equipment to work out holds true with this book. Now, there's genuinely no excuse'—**Sophie Choudry**, actor and singer

'Firstly, I *love* the title—it's "perfect"! The 10-minute workout *can* be done anywhere, and everyone is looking for a quick fix, so this should really work. What can I say about Yasmin except that she is truly a pioneer and is someone who is way ahead of her time. I vouch for her workouts—we all have been going to her over the years. I look up to her for fitness inspiration, and I think this book is another feather in her cap'—**Malaika Arora**, actor

'When I first visited Yasmin, I was quite vulnerable, and was struggling with finding new ways to get fitter. I also had a few knee issues, so I thought of Yasmin and decided to try Pilates. From the day we met, I found her positivity infectious, her energy levels high—important for a trainer—and her knowledge of fitness deep. Her approach to working out is scientific but at the same time, she also keeps the individual in mind. She not only trains you according to your body type but also as per your personality and mindset, and my workouts are tailored uniquely to my needs. Years ago, I had created a 25-minute programme to motivate people to start working out, and I think it is very important for people like Yasmin to come up with concepts like these. This book will not just help people get fitter but also improve their overall health; fitness is not just about how you look, but also about how you feel'—**Bipasha Basu**, actor

'I had the pleasure of training with Yasmin, and found her to be enthusiastic, encouraging, warm and very knowledgeable about human physiology. She was my introduction to Pilates, which I thoroughly enjoyed. I also appreciated her discipline, dedication and commitment towards helping those other than herself'—**Ishaan Khattar**, actor

'My association with Yasmin has been for as long as I have been working out. I started my fitness journey with her at the age of twenty-three when I got married. When I was pregnant with Ananya, Yasmin was also pregnant with her firstborn, and I would follow whatever she did. I worked out with her during both my pregnancies up to the ninth month, despite prevailing misconceptions at the time that one shouldn't work out during pregnancy. I think that doing so kept me very active and helped me lose my baby weight quickly and in a healthy manner. Since then, I have been working out with her intermittently. She pushes me to exercise as I am a very lazy person. I also get bored easily and to counter that, she creates workouts that are different every time, and that is what has made me last with her. She never gives up on me. Anyone else would have'—**Bhavana Pandey**, actor

'I love working out with Yasmin because she is learning and experimenting all the time. She practises what she preaches, inspiring others to follow her lead. I think that her idea of a 10-minute workout is great, as even a little movement every day goes a long way in the long run'—**Aaliyah Qureishi**, actor

'Yasmin is one of the few trainers who doesn't just focus on body transformation, but also on body recovery and overall fitness. Before I met her, I had many injuries, but she helped me recover. Her training programmes are both advanced and personalized, and no two workouts are the same. What I appreciate about her is that even after so many years, she is always learning. She regularly travels around the world to learn new techniques. She is a master in her field, but she still treats herself like a student. Yasmin taught me that fitness is not about hitting the gym for a couple of months; it is about falling in love with it. And it's not just about how you look from the outside but also your overall health. I feel that the 10-minute workouts will encourage more people to stay healthy. And with this book, there is no better way to start'—**Aayush Sharma**, actor

'I appreciate the time and effort Yasmin puts in to see the best results in her clients whether she trains them directly or not. She is always enquiring about their regime and diet and always has some positive input towards it. When I was training at her gym, I not only increased in strength, but also in flexibility, endurance, mobility and stamina. What makes YKBI different is their personalized approach towards general well-being and nutrition, which is a huge factor for any positive transformation'—**Aftab Shivdasani**, actor

'Yasmin was a friend before I started training with her and remains one of the best fitness trainers I have ever worked with. During a professional sports career, bodies develop wear and tear, and you sometimes need to train a bit differently to cope with the demands of playing at the international level. She trained me at a stage in my career where I needed to try something new. The first thing that strikes you about a good trainer is that they understand what an individual needs and design programmes accordingly and in that, and other ways, Yasmin is not just good, she is great! Pilates not only helped make a huge difference to my fitness levels and prolong my professional career but it also changed my life. With a book like this, you can improve your capabilities and your fitness levels. And no matter how fast-paced our lives are, there is simply no excuse *not* to find 10 minutes'—**Ajit Agarkar**, cricketer

'Not only does Yasmin have great energy, but she also achieves anything she sets her mind to. My body is in the best shape it has ever been only because of YKBI, and this book will help you get there too'—**Alizeh Agnihotri**, actor

'My entire family knows her, and mostly all have worked out with her, and there is no one who doesn't think highly of her. This book will be a game changer in the world of fitness brought to you by someone who has always worked hard to up her game'—**Alvira Agnihotri**, producer

'I started training with Yas almost twelve years ago and what I love about her the most is how she never drops the ball when it comes to fitness. She has amazing energy, knows how much to push you, and finds ways to work around the limits of your body. The whole concept of a 10-minute workout is amazing and will keep busy people active and fit. You can trust her advice; after all these years, she knows what she is talking about'—**Amrita Puri**, actor

'I have known Yasmin Karachiwala for more than thirty years, and I love the way she pushes me in our workout sessions but avoids injury at the same time. Her workouts are not repetitive, but they are challenging, and I love challenges. I credit her with my improved endurance; I can work out for longer times without getting tired. The concept of a 10-minute workout is a fabulous one, especially since the entire body is getting a workout with the exercises in this book! This is a great solution especially for those people who don't have the time to exercise'—**Anita Raaj**, actor

'I've known Yasmin—or Yasmin Body as I call her—since childhood. A fitness icon and role model, she has transformed people's bodies and with that their lives, and has helped so many celebrities achieve their goals, too. She's also helped many people recover from injuries, treated them and made them stronger. I remember going to her with my back issue. Within a few sessions, I could feel my back strengthening and things I found difficult to do—like bending, sitting for long periods, picking up stuff—I could do. She had identified which muscles were weak and what needed to be strengthened and even till today, I practice those simple exercises. The 10-minute stacks that she has designed with her trademark thoroughness can help you get great results'—**Arbaaz Khan**, actor and producer

'Having known Yasmin for over three decades now, I can vouch for the fact that Yasmin's workouts are part of her lifestyle. And that no matter where she is, she will always find a window for a quick workout. If you're with her, she will make you work out even on holiday! That said, her workouts are fun. She leads by example and through this book, she will make you aware of how easy it is to set aside 10 minutes of your day to stay healthy for life. She is a 10/10 when it comes to innovative routines, and this book of 10s reveals that side of her'—**Atul Agnihotri**, actor, director and producer

'Yasmin and I have known each other for over fifteen years, and the association that started professionally kept getting stronger as our clients got better. She, as a fitness expert, and I, as a physiotherapist, complement each other in rehabilitating our clients. Once I get them out of their agony, Yasmin gets them safely back to normal functioning in cases like knee replacements, ACL rehabilitation, disc derangements as well as shoulder, knee and ankle pain. She also further enhances the performance levels of her sports clients. I have also witnessed how painstakingly she designs customized workout programmes to suit her clients' unique needs, and I really admire her sincerity towards her clients. One word for this book—fabulous! It is simple and brilliantly written and is an exciting and handy guide to getting fit. In the time-poor world we live in, these quick 10-minute workouts will help rejuvenate us and make us feel so much better'—**Dr Hemakshi Basu**, physiotherapist

'It doesn't matter what challenge you throw at Yasmin—weight loss, weight gain, rehabilitation—she will find a solution that no one else can. The Perfect 10 is *perfect* for lives that are busy or for people who, despite their best intentions, can't seem to muster up the enthusiasm to stay fit'—**Isabelle Kaif**, actor

'She is as soft on the inside as her muscles are tough on the outside. And I have no doubt that if she has painstakingly designed and tested the 10-minute workouts in this book, that it will be a solid, workable solution'—**Jacqueline Fernandes**, actor

'I have had the privilege of knowing Yas for over a decade now, and she is a dear friend and a genuine soul. Yasmin's expertise in the field of fitness is matchless and her fun yet effective workouts, her discipline and her focus motivate her clients. She takes special care of all her clients and makes you understand that exercise should be a part of your daily regimen. Taking out time to exercise is hard in today's hectic life, and the 10-minute workout stacks will be very beneficial. Exercise improves blood circulation, enables micronutrients to reach the skin better, helps release toxins through sweat, and keeps your mind, body and skin radiant'—**Dr Jaishree Sharad**, cosmetic dermatologist

'My fitness journey began with Yas on her terrace gym in 2002, and she taught me everything I know about breath and form. I have never met anyone like her who lives such a wonderful lifestyle and makes it look so effortless. She's an inspiration, a friend and confidante. This book is a must for those who want access to Yasmin's vast knowledge about the body and health'—**Kim Sharma**, actor

'Lacking motivation or making excuses to not work out is common for most people. But it's hard to come up with excuses when all you need is 10 minutes of your day. As someone who swears by Yasmin's workouts, I can't wait for people to give this a shot! No more excuses'—**Kriti Kharbanda**, actor

'Not only does Yasmin have a perfect understanding of body mechanics, but she also customizes workouts based on need, mood and ability. The 10-minute workout is a wonderful concept for those who are time-poor or yet to discover the joy of lengthier routines. I eagerly look forward to this "perfect" companion for my busier days'—**Leena Tiwari**, industrialist

'It's such a cool concept and the idea of just 10 minutes a day to work out is great. I need to travel a lot because of my work; there's no schedule and my timings are so bizarre. Now I just need to carry this book, and I am set'—**Malvika Raaj**, actor

'Working out at YKBI has been one of the best decisions I have made till now. After dance, I never thought I would love any other form of exercise but thanks to Pilates and Yasmin, I do'—**Nataša Stanković Pandya**, dancer, model and actor

'Yas is just the best. I love her studio and her trainers. They are as invested as you in achieving your goals'—**Patralekhaa**, actor

'This book is a great way to take a break from the treadmill of life without using a treadmill. 10 minutes a day is all you need to start your journey to a fitter you, and once you start, you won't want to stop'—**Pooja Makhija**, nutritionist, biohacker and author

'I have been training with Yasmin for a decade now, and from being my trainer she is now my friend. What I admire about her the most is her consistency in her commitment towards her fitness, which has also had a huge impact on me. Her genius 10-minute stack hack is just the right amount of boost needed by the body and the mind but as you continue your fitness journey with this book, you might find that 10 minutes of Yas is not enough'—**Poorna Patel**, entrepreneur

'I love training with Yasmin. Her workout style is very effective in making you stronger, fitter and avoiding injury. I'm sure this book will help a lot of people very quickly as long as they remain consistent and follow the workouts'—**Preity Zinta**, actor

'I have known Yas for twenty years, and I have genuinely admired her for the balance she maintains between her profession and her family. As glamorous as she may appear, she has been an amazing daughter, daughter-in-law, mother and the most dedicated wife. Yas has a tremendous work ethic and her dedication to her clients is at another level. Her presence on Instagram has provided huge motivation for people from different fields. As a robotic and laparoscopic surgeon and a high-risk obstetrician, my fitness means a lot to me, and I thank Yas for setting my body right. Written by someone as experienced as her, this book is going to be a great source of inspiration and information'—**Dr Ranjana Dhanu**, robotic and laparoscopic surgeon, and OB/GYN

'Yasmin has carved a niche for herself and is a stalwart of the fitness world. Her clientele boasts of both celebrities and people from all walks of life. It will be great to read about tips that will motivate everyone'—**Raveena Tandon**, actor

'Everyone knows Yasmin, the Pilates Queen. However, I have had the good fortune, as her brother, to have a ringside view of her journey from a small room in her house dedicated to training her clients, to where she is today—at the forefront of the fitness industry in India. She is my only sibling on the planet but that is not the only reason she is special. She is a loving mother of two grown-up sons and a godmother to my two daughters, who lean on her for advice on everything in their lives. She is a perfectionist and is sharply focused on achieving results and today, she looks about twenty years younger than her chronological age because of her fitness regime, although she was least interested in exercise when she was younger! Many find Yas intimidating when they first meet her, because she comes across as a super-confident woman, which she is. However, she is also a softie, with a true heart of gold'—**Saif Qureishi**, entrepreneur and proud sibling

'My wife, Arathi, and I have been great admirers of Yasmin not just because she is a close friend, but also because of her passion for her work and for her ability to connect with people from all walks of life. She is not just beautiful on the outside but also has a wonderful heart, mind and soul. She is fun to be with, has tremendous positive energy and is outspoken and witty. While people are getting busier, the awareness of fitness is also simultaneously increasing, which is why the concept of a 10-minute workout will improve the lives of all who do it. Working out is not just about physical health but also about mental health'—**Shashi Kiran Shetty**, industrialist

'Yasmin Karachiwala forever looks stunning, so if she has innovated a 10-minute supersonic workout for supersonic busy people (or supersonic lazy people), I would blindly trust her book not only because she is a family friend, but also because of her experience, knowledge, and scientific approach towards well-being'—**Sohail Khan**, actor and producer

'When I came to Yasmin, I was physically and mentally broken, but thanks to her, my body transformed. I think these 10-minute stacks would be very beneficial for building your fitness, which is not just about looking good, but very necessary for dealing with life's challenges. Fitness makes you a warrior'—**Srisha Reddy**, former tennis player

'Yasmin is an institution in herself of self-care, health, nutrition, beauty and fitness in India. There is no stopping her and that is because of her dogged determination to excel in everything she does. Whether the client is sixty or sixteen years old, she works her magic to suit the individual. What better timing than now for this amazing book, which comes out at a time of global uncertainty about health, and I am sure it will reach out to millions who struggle to find the time or the inclination to work out. Thanks to Yasmin, I too can now work out anywhere, which means, I can't make excuses (wink)! She genuinely inspires me, and I am sure this book will inspire many others to look at fitness from a whole new perspective'—**Vaibhavi Merchant**, choreographer

'In today's world, when people (like me!) complain that they don't have enough time to work out because of their busy schedules, that will no longer be the case because of this book! And since this book has been created by an expert like Yasmin, you should blindly trust her and go for it. Everyone should have their own copy. I want to thank Yasmin for writing this book, and I look forward to keeping it with me all the time'—**Sunil Grover**, actor and comedian

# THE PERFECT 10

## 10-MINUTE WORKOUTS
## YOU CAN DO ANYWHERE

# YASMIN
# KARACHIWALA

*with* GAYATRI PAHLAJANI

EBURY
PRESS

An imprint of Penguin Random House

EBURY PRESS

USA | Canada | UK | Ireland | Australia
New Zealand | India | South Africa | China | Singapore

Ebury Press is part of the Penguin Random House group of companies
whose addresses can be found at global.penguinrandomhouse.com

Published by Penguin Random House India Pvt. Ltd
4th Floor, Capital Tower 1, MG Road,
Gurugram 122 002, Haryana, India

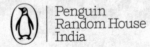

First published in Ebury Press by Penguin Random House India 2023

ISBN 9780143457619

Typeset in Minion Pro by Manipal Technologies Limited, Manipal
Printed at Thomson Press India Ltd, New Delhi

*Dedicated to*
*my parents*

# Contents

**Part One: Where We Are. What We Need**
*Why we are the way we are, and what we can do about it*

**Part Two: The Workouts**
*Discover the world of fitness 10 minutes at a time*
*Also included are bonus exercises for various*
*health conditions including what we're all*
*guilty of—bad posture*

# Prologue

## *Fingers versus Bodies*

If you're reading this book, chances are that you have typed and tapped your way to its purchase. Chances also are that you have typed and tapped your way to other things today. Never in the history of human existence has so much been accomplished by moving so little. Buying groceries, running businesses, fighting wars—these are now being mobilized more by fingers, not bodies. With cheerful gloom, I predict that in addition to the other troubles we may face as a planet, this is the war of the future—that between our fingers and our bodies. And if our fingers win, it means only one thing—our bodies lose.

Bad things happen when our bodies are not being used for the purposes they are designed for. Obesity, diabetes, cardiac disease, cancer—they all come a-pinging. Our bodies were designed to move—to fight enemies, to conquer territories, to *survive*. Can you imagine if the first man sat on his gluteus maximus? The enemy—wild animals, crazy birds, whatever—approaches him but he's preoccupied with sending flirty texts to the first woman? Uh-oh, too late. End of humanity.

We are here *because* of our instincts for movement. This descent into our couches is relatively new. It's only in the last century or so that we've had to *think* of exercising. Lethargy is suddenly an epidemic, sitting is suddenly the new smoking, but the warning signs have been in place for some time. The future of a life without movement is a future we are already beginning to live in. So many diseases are caused partly or wholly due to a fundamental lack of activity and while we have cures, they do not always restore a pre-disease quality of life. Either way, do we really want it to get that far?

The problem with Fitness—and here I use a capital F—is that it is its own enemy. And, that enemy is its reputation. A reputation that has been harnessed by a multi-billion-dollar culture that favours speed over well-being, aesthetic over health, sweat over efficiency. There is little or no reward for incremental gain. Fitness *looks* hard. Weight maintenance *looks* difficult. It is a culture that has normalized half-truths for so long and so deeply that these have become part of our conditioning and discouraged us from seeking out our own path to better health.

Normalize this: fitness is *easy*. This book will show you that all it takes is *10 minutes* a day to start that journey and it is packed with exercise plans, movement ideas and lifestyle changes.

Get up. Move with me. And see how your body and your life changes.

Don't let those fingers win.

This book has been divided into three parts. You can, of course, head straight to the workout section in **Part Two**, BUT we would recommend that you read the chapters in the order they have been written, skim through the 10-Minute Workout Stacks contents page on page 77 to shortlist your first set of workouts, finish the rest of the book, and then go back to **Part Two** and start exercising. Each chapter has useful tips and insights based on my thirty years of fitness experience, so it may help to read them before you begin working out with this book.

We are also extremely excited to announce that EVERY exercise in The Perfect 10: 10-Minute Workouts You Can Do Anywhere *has video instruction. ALL 10-minute stacks (and warm-up and cool-down workouts) have been designed and shot exclusively for you, and wherever possible, we have also provided easier, modified versions of the exercises. To access the videos, all you have to do is:*

1. *Scan the QR code.*
2. *Select the 10-minute workout and exercise with me—a virtual one-on-one personal training session for every exercise in this book!*

The written workout instructions—which is why this book is so thick!—are simply backup options in case you have weak Wi-Fi or mobile phone connectivity or don't have access to your phone.

# Foreword

The first time I met Yasmin, I squeezed her arms. To be clear, this is not the way I normally behave. I mean, I don't usually meet people for the first time by squeezing them. But I couldn't help both notice and admire the sleekness of her arms.

*'I want these,'* I remember saying.

*'Three weeks,'* she promised.

And that was the beginning of our journey.

For most of my career, I have worked with Yasmin on all my fitness goals. We have worked together on most of my films and were able to achieve whatever different fitness targets we had for that required role. We adapted our workouts to suit the objective, and played with a mix of Pilates, functional training, high intensity interval training (HIIT), aerobics, multi-functional training (MFT), among other things that made a big difference, sometimes in a very short space of time. She didn't just help me achieve every target I set out to achieve; she worked with me on building a solid foundation of muscle on which I could construct any fitness dream.

With affection and without bias, I can say that Yasmin is one of the best fitness trainers we have. I see evidence of this in her commitment to excellence, her deep knowledge of her craft, her consistent investment in updating her skill set and her insatiable (read: insane) need to challenge her body. There is an age gap of over ten years between us, and I mention it precisely because it is a huge inspiration to see someone older than me, who is fitter than many half her age. It is easy to get complacent at her level and she understands both the benefits of reinvention as well as the risks of stagnation. You can tell that she wants to be the best at what she does. And that she wants the best for her clients too.

I am an actor, an entrepreneur and now a wife. With every role I take on, the busier it gets, and it is so easy to succumb to the attitude of skipping a workout because I don't have a 'perfect' 45 minutes for the gym. *The Perfect 10: 10-Minute Workouts You Can Do Anywhere* has been written for the thousands of people Yas has met along the way who, like me, have the intention, but don't always have the time. Or for those who saw fitness as something unattainable—a thing of fascination, but not participation. Or for those who wanted to get fitter but didn't know where to begin. To them I say that I know how they feel, but we have to start *somewhere*.

*The Perfect 10* is that somewhere. Its '10-minute stack' approach introduces—for the first time in India—a flexible way of working out that expands (or contracts) to suit the time *you* have available, with modifications for those entering the world of fitness for the first time. You'll also find advice on nutrition, sleep, hydration, pre-workout recipes and how to break the dreaded fitness plateau. But I think its biggest benefit lies in the message it carries with its format: that *consistency* is better than perfection. That doing something even for *10* minutes a day is better than waiting for a perfect time to do *more later*. That while developing strength or stamina is crucial, equally important is building the fitness *habit*. And that if you just make that commitment to yourself, everything else you want will follow.

No two fitness journeys are the same, and perfection is a matter of opinion. What I would say to anyone who is starting their fitness journey is always start from where *you* are. And if you keep it consistent, you'll get to where you never thought you'd be. I speak from experience.

Katrina Kaif
Mumbai, 2022

# Introduction

## *An Opening Note by Yasmin*

As a child, I was many things but, 'fit' was not one of them. My older brother, the golden child, was a star athlete and a star student and I felt that it was important to bring balance to the family, so I was neither. There would be no challenge for my parents if both their children were overachievers, I thought.

No one was more surprised than I was when I chose fitness for a living because I spent my childhood resisting its call. My mother, the yoga nut, tried unsuccessfully to convince me to take the bus with her for classes. My father, a known pounder of the Mahalaxmi racecourse track, struggled in vain to get me to do more than quarter of a round. In school, they tried to suck me into sports, but I was too clever for them. I signed up for shot put and javelin because I could do the most by moving the least.

But it was my best friend, or rather her need to impress a boy, that was my first proper introduction to fitness. There was a 2-for-1 deal at a swanky new health club and she blackmailed me into going with her, because that way we would each pay only half. Since I didn't want to upset her, I agreed. On our first day, while she confidently strode towards the weights section, I followed a small herd going into the aerobics studio. In my head, I was a fantastic dancer. Aerobics would be a breeze, I thought.

It was more of a hurricane. When the class went right, I went left. I was consistently south-east to their north-west and there wasn't one bum that hadn't met my foot. With the absence of any self-awareness, I also started coming early to reserve my spot right in front of the class. When someone justifiably asked me if I could go to the back because, in her words, I was 'doing rubbish', she unleashed my stubborn streak. I would go to the back but I was determined to earn my spot in front of the class again, just so I could prove them wrong.

Nostrils flared and shoulders squared with a new sense of purpose, my feet eventually stopped connecting with other people's bodies. I must have become considerably better because one day, and much to my surprise, the instructor called and asked me to take over her class:

> *Hi Yasmin!*
> Hi.
> *Can you take the class tomorrow? I'm not well. I'll tell you where the music is.*
> How do I take the class?
> *Play the music and do what you remember.*

Armed with those detailed instructions, I took the class. My brain seemed to be disconnected from my body. Someone who looked like me and talked like me seemed to know all the steps. She gave clear instructions. She corrected form and posture. She clapped. She cheered. She led. She was no longer 'doing rubbish'. At the end of the class, the same people who I had once injured, applauded, although I suspect it was more out of relief. The class was over, and nobody died. That day, I learnt three things:

1. When I put my mind to it, I can stop kicking people.
2. When someone tells me I can't do something, I see it as an invitation to prove them wrong.
3. I love telling people what to do.

When the instructor got pregnant, I started taking her afternoon classes. I also started getting compensated for it, so it became my first paid job at eighteen. It still wasn't a career choice for me at that time, but just something I was doing along with attending college, taking exams and hanging out with friends. And while fitness eventually evolved into a more serious career, my ambition was cemented on the back of an incident that changed my life.

In October 1990, the same best friend, who talked me into the gym membership, had a party at her house. But just before the party started, she called at the last minute to say that things were not okay at home and asked me not to leave. My parents came back from dinner, surprised to see me because they thought I had already left. We all turned in for the night. There would be no party to go to today.

About half an hour later, the phone rang. It was my friend again. Things had settled, and she asked whether I could come. Since my parents already knew I was going out for the night, I drove to her house, which was 5 minutes away. She lived in a bungalow with the family rooms upstairs and the living areas below. When I entered, the living room was set up for a celebration, but things were quiet. We were a much smaller party now, about five of us, and we sat chatting amongst ourselves.

I don't remember how much time had elapsed; it could have been minutes or maybe more when there was a loud noise, and suddenly bullets were being fired at us. My best friend got shot, and fell face forward on a bed, followed by her mother, who crumpled in a heap on the floor. Others got shot at too, but, somehow, I managed to escape. Since I was the only one left who could drive and who wasn't injured, I tore out of the house, unlocked my car with shaking hands and rushed to a nearby hospital to get an ambulance. As soon as I pulled up and got out, I started screaming for help. They told me that if it was a shootout, then it was a police case and that I needed to go to a public hospital, which was 5 minutes away. By the time I managed to get the ambulance, it was too late for my best friend and her mother. They died on the way to the hospital.

I remember calling my father from a public phone outside the hospital, howling, saying words that didn't mean anything to him, like 'shooting', 'fire', 'gun' and 'dead'. He obviously couldn't understand what I was saying. I had to tell him where I was and by the time my parents rushed to the hospital, I was steeling myself to give statements to the police.

Mental health today is not what it was in 1990, and there were few resources to help you heal from a tragedy like this. For years I felt guilty, and I didn't know why. I graduated the following year in a haze. Memories of my best friend were everywhere, from where she sat in college, the lanes we walked, to the streets we drove around. I wanted to leave my old life for a while. Ordinarily, my conservative Muslim family wouldn't have let me do that, but they could see how much this incident affected me. And it was because of this that I was allowed to go to the United States to study aerobics, which further cemented my determination to make something of it.

The American fitness scene in 1991 was way ahead of anything I had ever seen back home. The fitness industry in India was still in its infancy—most instructors were using Jane Fonda's video home system (VHS) workouts to learn and teach their classes. There was little understanding of the notion of *studying* fitness, which came to India much later. That said, people were just happy to exercise; aerobics was fun, it was choreographed like a dance, and it really caught on. There were a smattering of well-known dance studios, one of which I rented to conduct my aerobics classes when I returned to India in 1992.

I was a total rebel back then, so when I was introduced to my future husband, Minhaz, by a common friend of both our parents, I decided to wear torn jeans—not the fashion statement they are now—and a jacket, for our first meeting. My brother saw me as I was leaving, and said that I looked like someone who played for a wedding band, and not a good one. My mother was appropriately horrified, but I had a plan. I was determined to look as hideous as I could, because I believed that if someone could like me at my worst, they would love me at my best.

Minhaz and I hit it off from the start. He was, and remains, an introvert to my extrovert, the calm to my crazy and the order to my chaos. When we got married, I moved to his house in Cuffe Parade, in south Mumbai. Marriage only made me work harder to keep my ambition going. From doing step classes to teaching English to toddlers as a preschool teacher, I spent those early years experimenting and learning, while strapping my firstborn to the back seat and driving almost daily to Bandra, a fifty-kilometre round-trip. My husband used to joke that I spent more on petrol than I earned, but I didn't care.

After my second baby, I became a personal trainer (PT) and went from house to house to train, but I soon found that my clients didn't take their workouts seriously. There was always something more important to attend to—a ringing doorbell, a cook, a spouse looking for a sock—so I got my PT clients to come to my newly set-up home gym after we moved to Bandra, to free them from distractions. Around that time, my celebrity clients also started to trickle in, starting with my home gym and then later my studio—Kareena Kapoor Khan was my first, followed by Urmila Matondkar, Kim Sharma, Malaika Arora, Karisma Kapoor, Amrita Arora, Neha Dhupia, Hrithik Roshan, Arjun Rampal, Kunal Kapoor, Ajit Agarkar, Zaheer Khan and latterly Katrina Kaif, Alia Bhatt, Deepika Padukone, Hardik Pandya, Sophie Choudry, Kriti Sanon, Kiara Advani, Vaani Kapoor, Bipasha Basu, Preity Zinta, Huma Qureshi, Sonakshi Sinha, Ananya Panday, Patralekhaa, Sohail Khan, Aayush Sharma, Sonam Kapoor Ahuja and Jacqueline Fernandes, among others.

My first studio was in an apartment in Bandra, in the adjoining building in the society. The day after I started operations, the building society took me to court. They knew that I was starting a gym—it is hard to hide the unloading of a treadmill or the unpacking of a training bench—and I thought we had the permissions, but they chose to issue a notice after I had invested everything I had.

I decided to fight the case and went to the cooperative court alone every fortnight using the abundance of free time I had in between raising two boys, managing a house, training clients, focusing on my own fitness and working full-time. We won the case in the cooperative court but the society then took me to the High Court and sent notices to all my celebrity clients, by when I gave up because of the relentlessness of it all. I sold the gym and started a new one, which did very well for nine years, after which we moved into our current flagship property in Bandra. We've expanded our operations and at the time of going to press, we have franchises in Delhi, Gurugram, Dubai, Dhaka, Ahmedabad and Indore.

None of this would have been possible without the support of two families—the one I was born into and the one I married into. My mother always told me that if I treated my in-laws like my in-laws, I would always be a daughter-in-law, but if I considered them parents, I would be their daughter. As I write this, my mother-in-law is stitching a bikini for me and my mother remains as appalled by this as she was the day I met Minhaz in torn jeans.

Fitness has changed since the first time I entered a gym. There are many more options available but the biggest shift I find is that more people acknowledge the need for it, have more conversations around it and are more clued in about trends. They are also more attuned to their internal workings, and are open-minded about seeking alternate ways to deliver what their bodies need.

But with Instagram, social media, video calls and selfies, our culture has also become more visually-oriented and clients are more conscious than ever about how they look. I would say about a third of my clients work out for reasons other than looking good, but most are motivated by signs of tangible, visual progress. What remains the same—and what I would like to change—is an unhealthy preoccupation with numbers. For a truly fit, happy and beautiful life, all you need to do is show up for your body every single day, enjoy what you do, resist shortcuts, and not be obsessed by how much you weigh. That is when the magic truly unfolds.

Yasmin Karachiwala
Mumbai, 2022

# PART ONE: WHERE WE ARE. WHAT WE NEED

1

# Fingers 1, Bodies 0

*Exploring our descent into couches and how our environment conspires against us to discourage movement*

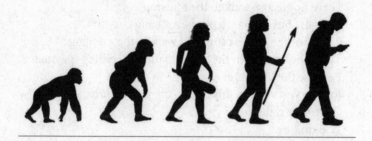

Before us there were early prototypes of us, discovering new ways to make life easier. Evidence suggests that Homo Habilis, who existed about 2.4 million years ago, may have shaped tools out of stones.[*] Homo Erectus, who populated the earth about 1.9 million years ago, used fire to cook and even perhaps protect themselves.[†] Not to be outdone, we Homo Sapiens started to invent ways to make our lives more efficient and have been gloriously successful at it.

---

[*] 'Homo Habilis,' *Smithsonian National Museum of Natural History*, accessed 8 December 2022, https://humanorigins.si.edu/evidence/human-fossils/species/homo-habilis.

[†] 'Homo Erectus,' *Smithsonian National Museum of Natural History*, accessed 8 December 2022, https://humanorigins.si.edu/evidence/human-fossils/species/homo-erectus.

From the invention of the wheel to the airplane to the smartphone, the descent into our couches has been all but inevitable.

Cut to the twenty-first century, and we have been so good at this that we now live in what I like to call a 'movement-repellent' world. We are able to do a lot more with our time, but exercise doesn't seem to be one of the things. But before we beat ourselves up, we need to understand that it happened without us even realizing it. Here is an example from not too long ago.

## Paying the Phone Bill

**c. 1990**
1. Leave home and walk to the bus stop.
2. Take the bus to the telephone exchange.
3. Get off at the nearest stop and walk to the exchange.
4. Take the stairs to the floor handling billing payments. Because the lift is broken.
5. Realize you've been directed to the wrong floor.
6. Get to the right floor.
7. Wait in line.
8. Pay the bill.
9. Walk back to the bus stop.
10. Take the bus home.
11. Walk home from the bus stop.

**Calories burned:** 200–300, depending on body type.

**Now**
1. Pick up phone to read text.
2. Pay the bill on phone.

**Calories burned:** Less than 20, assuming you have a very heavy pair of thumbs.

**Total unburnt calorie deficit:** 200–300.

Now, add this deficit to the lines you didn't stand at the bank, the walking you didn't do at the store or the distance you didn't cover in the grocery aisle. Activities that burned one or two thousand calories a week have now been virtually eliminated. It takes 3500 calories burned to lose a pound of body weight, and it is the weight we would have otherwise lost or maintained had we been doing what we had always been doing. Physical activity is sneakily making its way out of our lives and obesity levels are only rising.[*] India is now one of the top five countries in terms of obese populations.[†] With all this going on, why don't we exercise more?

I was getting my hair trimmed once and I thought I'd ask my stylist precisely this question because I am a fun person to be with. He spent a considerable length of time telling me why he *didn't* exercise, systematically listing all the obstacles he found along the way. It mirrored scores of conversations I have had with people, including my clients, about their fitness routines and, from these, a few things have become clear about why we struggle with getting fitter. For starters,

**Fitness is now an errand of its own.**
**A thing to do, a box to tick.**

It is not that we cannot move or don't want to. We subscribe to a work culture that not only asks the individual to sacrifice more of their personal time, but we begrudge ourselves even the little time spent on our well-being. Anything that is associated with

---

[*] 'Forecasting the prevalence of overweight and obesity in India to 2040,' *National Library of Medicine*, accessed 12 October 2022, https://www.ncbi.nlm.nih.gov/pmc/articles/PMC7039458/.

[†] 'NFHS-5: Indians are getting fatter - and it's a big problem,' *BBC News*, accessed 14 October 2022, https://www.bbc.com/news/world-asia-india-61558119.

care of the self has to come *after* making a living, *after* taking care
of your family or *after* spending time with friends.

The environment doesn't make it easy for you either.
Imagine, for example, a conversation with your boss asking for a
day off to trek in the mountains.

Scenario A (The Truth)
*Could I take tomorrow off?*
Why?
*It's been rough at work lately, and I thought I'd reconnect with
nature.*
<long pause>
Can you take off after the presentation? <which is weeks away>
It's a bad time.
*I understand.*

Scenario B (Complete Lies)
*Could I take tomorrow off?*
Why?
*My mother is not feeling too good, and I may have to take her to
the hospital.*
Absolutely. I understand.

In other words, most well-oiled corporate machines legitimize
time off usually in the most emergent circumstances, forgetting
that from time-to-time human beings need a little oiling too.

## Fitness is confrontation

Fitness in its current form is an oftentimes unpleasant
confrontation between you and your body. Its twenty-first
century format is goal-based, number-driven, intensive and
at many times, joyless. It is designed to make you face the
limitations of your body, to *push* you—whatever that means—

to inadvertently remind you about your weaknesses and your follies. While you *do* need some amount of encouragement to expand your capacity, many current programmes are sprints, not marathons. They have become new sources of stress because you didn't set the pace.

## Fitness is a destination

Another of the more frequent attitudes I encounter is that once a goal has been achieved—say six-pack abdominals or a number on the scale or better blood pressure (BP) readings—that is the *end*. The destination has been reached, and work no longer has to be done. The idea that fitness has to be continually maintained through more *fitness* comes as a surprise to many. Fitness is a journey with *multiple* destinations that change, the fitter you become.

## Fitness is thinness

I idolized the legendary trainer Pervez Mistry, who was kind enough to mentor me early in my career. I would work out at his gym for hours, follow every instruction and take notes like he was the rockstar and I was his groupie. I thought I was a gold-star student until one day he said, 'Did you know that you're a fat-thin person?' I shook my head. 'You are a thin person on the outside,' he continued, 'but are fat on the inside.' I nodded, now feeling annoyed on the inside. Of course, he was right, like he always was. He meant that I had not built enough muscle yet and if I wanted to be a fitness trainer, I needed to be fit *myself* by building muscle and shedding fat.

Raise your hand if you have said, heard or thought the following: *You are so thin. Why do you need to work out?* Another hurdle to getting fitter is that people equate fitness with thinness and that is simply not true. When clients stand on the Body

Composition machine, they are usually shocked by how much body fat they have, even though they are underweight. This is common for us Indians—we overwhelmingly have what are called 'Skinny Fat' bodies, which are low in weight and high in fat. And bodies high in fat usually mean one thing—they are low in muscle.

But why is it a problem if your body is low in muscle? The best way I can explain it is that fat and muscle share the same real estate which is, of course, your body. A gram of fat and a gram of muscle both weigh a gram, but the gram of

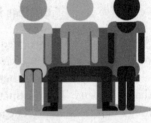

muscle takes up far lesser square footage. You would think that they would both live in harmony, but that isn't the case. Fat is like the manspreader in the picture, and the more space it gets, the more space over time it will occupy. The other people trying to squeeze into the seat? That's poor little muscle, getting squashed.

The more fat cells you have, the more efficient your body gets at storing fat. The better your body gets at storing fat, the more fat cells it acquires. And the more fat cells it acquires, the more square footage *you* acquire. There's only one way you can stop this cycle, and that's by building more muscle—it not only takes up less real estate, making you look sleeker, but also burns more calories at rest than fat does, keeping your weight down.

## Fitness is related only to the body

*So* many people forget that fitness improves your mental agility, your reflexes, your stamina, your sleep, your performance at work, your sex life, your view of the world and your mood, and is prescribed as adjunct therapy to pretty much all mental health illnesses and many physical ones. And that's just off the top of my head.

I remember a client who came to me in some degree of frustration because she was working out for three months and still had not lost any weight. So I asked her the following:

Do you feel better? *Yes.*
Do you sleep better? *Yes.*
Have you lost inches? *Yes, many.*
Are you more focused at work? *Yes.*
Do you look better in your clothes than you did before? *Yes.*
So, what's the problem? *I am not losing weight.*

Her body fat composition revealed a significant increase in muscle over those three months but as it weighs more than fat, the net result on the scale in terms of weight loss was zero. She eventually did lose kilos on the scale, but not before muscle planted its flag.

Joseph Pilates used to say that you are as young as your spine is flexible. Or simply, your age is determined not by years but by how fit you are. Most people have an actual age and a metabolic age. There are some sixty-year-olds who have the fitness of forty-year-olds and I have seen many in my business who are in their twenties but their metabolic age is double their biological age. Working out is not just about looking good or feeling good, it adds years to your life and, as they say, life to your years.

But, in the battle between fingers and bodies, the fingers win, because given the current fitness environment, few people *want* to exercise even if they have the time. I mean, who likes stress? Who likes to be reminded of their weaknesses? Who wants to make a lifelong commitment? People have to work out but more often, they don't *want* to. *Have to* is not the same as *want*. *Have to* is not a great pitch. *Have to* doesn't bring you joy. *Have to* doesn't allow you to stay on track.

The best way to be fit for life is to increase the *want* factor.

## Increasing the *Want* Factor—Finding Your Fitness Happiness

Finding your fitness happiness is very important if you want to make a lifelong commitment to fitness because you cannot sustain something that doesn't give you joy. Increasing the *want* factor is about identifying your exercise personality and customizing an active lifestyle for yourself. And while many people like the pushing, the shouting, the yelling, the looking-into-the-mirror-and-pumping, not everyone does. As there are people, there are fitness personalities, and identifying yours could be key to you sticking to a routine and giving yourself something to look forward to.

Here are a few I've found. Nod if any of these apply to you.

### The Steadfasts

The Steadfasts are those who like to do what is required of their workouts—not too much, not too little, just the right amount. They want a trainer who won't let them slack off but won't push them too hard. They're regular and like their workouts. These people have identified what they want in a fitness routine and are happiest with small shake-ups in their routine, but don't like to be alarmed. They like to come in at least three times a week for an hour and for them I usually recommend splitting their workouts into three parts with progressive changes in weights and repetitions—Day 1 (Legs and Shoulders), Day 2 (Back and Biceps) and Day 3 (Chest and Triceps). For variety, I often also suggest circuit training every alternate week, as well as mixing up the body parts and trying newer exercises.

## The Overachievers

Every gym has a few of these—those who seem to 'live' there. Nothing stands between them and achieving their goals, and they want to be constantly challenged. Their workouts are an obsession and they expect a great deal from their instructors. They are best suited for more demanding programmes like boot camps, powerlifting, kickboxing and the like. For them, I would only ask that they listen to their bodies by making sure they identify good pain from bad, and take more rest days.

## The Dreamers

Bless them, but there are also those that want the results, but don't want to work for it. They want a six-pack, but don't want to diet. Or their friend lost weight and they want to be exactly like them even though they have completely different body types. Or they want to start a fitness programme with a high degree of complexity without understanding that their bodies aren't ready for it yet, and so they have to be dissuaded or pushed. These kinds of clients usually have a high drop-out rate and dissatisfaction with most exercise programmes. For these people, I gently recommend reality.

## The Big Dippers

These people dip into everything, from Zumba to Pilates to yoga to boxing. They need constant stimulation and regular shake-ups in their schedule. They are also, in my experience, those that have bursts of fitness followed by lulls, and are a target group prone to high drop-out rates. For these people, I recommend a studio class with varying workouts or multiple fitness programmes.

## The Sports Hobbyists

Regular swimmers, golfers, squash players, tennis enthusiasts, runners, cyclists, basketball and football players are people who see their physical activity more as a hobby, and for them the *want* factor is already in-built. These people usually have lifelong commitments to their physical activities and derive great pleasure from them. For this target group, I suggest doing Pilates at least once a week.

## The Groupies

These people love working out in groups or need an exercise buddy. They don't like walking alone, for example, and they also are not as motivated if they are doing it alone. For them, I usually suggest group classes like Zumba, Pilates and dancing, but only if they focus more on the workout and not talking amongst themselves.

## The Goalies

Then there are those who come in with a goal, like getting fit for a wedding, losing baby weight or preparing for a film role. Once the objective has been achieved, they tend to taper off their programmes, until they find a new target. For them, I recommend setting a more sustainable goal—that of consistency. My clients Deepika Padukone and Katrina Kaif, for example, have made fitness part of their lifestyle, work on their bodies throughout the year, and are 'shot-ready' even when they're not shooting.

## The Walkers

You see them everywhere. Mornings and evenings, on promenades, roads, parks and beaches, pounding the surface and getting their daily dose of fresh air. Walking is one of the best exercises anyone can do but the Walkers often feel they're not seeing results. I usually advise them to mix up their walking routines—climb uphill, jog in phases or change their route, which will push their bodies out of their comfort zones. If you do the same thing day after day, your body is no longer being challenged.

## The Reluctants

These include kids forced by their parents, husbands forced by their wives, wives forced by their doctors, or people who don't exercise at all forced by an old photograph of theirs which shocked them. In these workouts, no one is having fun. The kid doesn't want to move, the husband is unenthusiastic and the wife is moving like some tortoises on some beaches. This segment tends to taper off their workouts entirely with big breaks in between. In addition to venture capitalists and banks, the Reluctants are also the biggest funders of the fitness industry because they pay and rarely show up. I have often wanted to name a treadmill after them. For them, I recommend starting slow with workouts they truly enjoy.

I find that most people are a combination of at least two of the above—I've encountered Steadfast Walkers, Overachieving Groupies, Overachieving Goalies, and so on. Some instinctively understand their exercise personalities, while others have to kiss many frogs before they find their perfect match. Either way:

**To find your fitness happiness is to find your fitness personality.**

## The Time Poor

This encompasses all of the above, and this is why *The Perfect 10: 10-Minute Workouts You Can Do Anywhere* has been written. It has challenges for the Overachievers, workouts for the Steadfasts, variations for the Big Dippers, results for the Goalies, workouts for the Sports Hobbyists who can't step out, and provides enough of an incentive for even the most Reluctant. What is 10 minutes after all?

Bodies are wonderful, magical and responsive things. They respond to neglect, a poorly-designed workout, a well thought-out plan, fresh fruit, rotting meat, strength training, cardio workouts, inconsistent practice, good nourishment, water and sunlight, all in different ways. If people start looking at fitness differently, they would live longer, healthier lives with fewer problems that hold them back from their careers and their lives. The side effect is, of course, to look and feel the best they ever have.

The more consistent you are with your fitness, the fitter you get. The fitter you get, the fitter you *want* to get and the fitter you *should* get, because the battle of tomorrow may not even be between fingers and bodies. The future of technology is exciting but predicts only further relinquishment of physical activity. Smart watches are replacing phones. We are now wearing technology. We are now speaking to technology. While the future of organic fitness does not look good, that should not deter you from a world that I promise you is unexpectedly joyful and immensely rewarding.

And it starts with just 10 minutes.

2

# SMASH*N Your Fitness Goals

## *Six key fitness rules.*
## *And only one of them is exercise*

Of the people that many find annoying are the ones who seem to eat what they want without seemingly gaining any weight. We stare at them over our salads as they order fries—*'Could you make them extra crispy, please?'*—and quietly burn with envy. Extra crisply, of course.

Since the start of my career over thirty years ago, I have seen more bodies than most undertakers and I can tell you that while it is true that some people start out with more naturally efficient metabolisms, age is a great leveller. Most people who infuriate us with their lean physiques consistently work on them, fries or no fries, consciously or unconsciously. What is also true is that most people think that there are only two aspects to fitness—diet and exercise—but they would only be partially correct. There are no less than *six* determinants and if you're not seeing the results you want, chances are you are not doing all six.

The fastest way I remember these six key players is to call it the SMASH*N approach, not just because it's the best way to smash your fitness goals but also because it is the universal basis to look, well, smashing. You are welcome.

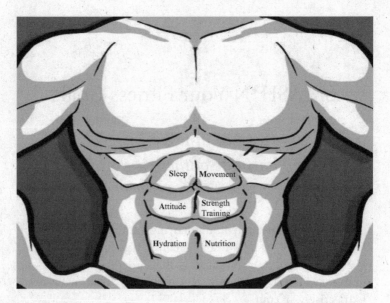

The SMASH*N Approach

## SMASH*N YOUR FITNESS GOALS—SLEEP

The ABC of fitness starts with the ZZZs. Sleep is when your body does the all-important work of healing from the natural wear and tear of the day. Not only is it one of the foundations of physiological efficiency—from cognition to immunity to metabolism to movement—it also regulates the appetite, which means it regulates your diet and consequently, your weight.

Most people know how much they need to sleep and when they're short on it. Trainers can also tell the difference by how you perform:

*z z z Z*

*z*

'One. Two. Three.'                    'One... Two ... Three.'

If you find yourself struggling despite working out at the same weight or difficulty level, you're probably just tired. When you're rested, you've also rested your muscles, which are then able to perform better. Sleep makes you stronger.

*z z z Z*

*z*

'Good form, GOOD FORM.'        'Bend your knees, don't arch
                               your back, neck straight, blah,
                               blah, blah ...'

How attentive you are during your workouts is sometimes inversely proportional to how much noise your trainer is making. If your trainer demands that you pay attention, is constantly checking your form or is just more vocal in general, chances are that it is not because they are having a bad day but because you are. Sleep deprivation affects both your ability to focus on your workout and maintain proper form, which, in turn, increases your chances of injury.

$z^z z^Z Z$

z

*'I'm ready.'*                          *'Gimme a MINUTE.'*

Recovery time is that little break during a workout—a walk during a run, a pause between weight training, a low-impact section in a group class. It is taken to ensure that your body achieves homeostasis, defined as 'any self-regulating process by which an organism tends to maintain stability while adjusting to conditions that are best for its survival.'* By slowing down your heart rate, recovery times allow your body to adjust to the intensity of a workout without overwhelming it. Tired bodies take longer to recover for the next part of a workout and when they do, they rarely approach it with the same intensity.

That said, I applaud my clients' determination in coming for their workouts despite being sleep-deprived; I've been there. But it is precisely from personal experience I say that without adequate rest, they will invest both time and money without deriving *value*. Do inform your trainer that you're tired or if you're not feeling it; they'll take your workout down a notch. If they don't, change your trainer. No one knows your body better than you.

It is also important to mention here that not everyone can—and should—work out at the same time. Few things shatter my peace more than an early morning workout. I am happy to train other early birds, but don't take me down with you. After trial and error, I have discovered that 11.30 a.m. is my sweet spot

---

* 'Homeostasis physiology,' *Britannica*, accessed 12 October 2022, https://www.britannica.com/science/homeostasis.

and starting even an hour earlier can diminish my performance. People often ask me what the best time is to work out, and I often say that the best time to work out is the best time for *you*.

For a good night's sleep, try these:

1. *Sleep and wake at about the same time:* If you play too fast and loose with your bedtimes, your body finds it hard to settle down into a rhythm, which it needs to work better.
2. *Work out to pass out:* A good workout is also designed to tire you out, setting the stage for good, sound sleep. But avoid exercising too close to bedtime. Exercise releases stimulating hormones like adrenalin, which pump you up. There is an entirely different set of hormones to wind you down, which is why your body will resist sleep until they take over.
3. *Avoid stimulants too close to bedtime:* Coffee, tea, and screen time, all interfere with the natural circadian rhythm of your body. Resist the urge to 'revenge scroll' or switch to decaf in the second half of the day. If you find it hard to drift off, try an analogue reading device—otherwise known as books—for some me-time that doesn't interfere with your ZZZ-time.
4. *Practice good bedtime habits:* A soothing drink, a warm bath, relaxing music, deep breathing are all sleep-inducing habits that can be introduced before bedtime. Also, do make sure your room is dark so that your body produces more melatonin.

I would advise those who are very short on sleep—less than six hours for me, but it can vary from person to person—to not undertake heavy workouts. You can go for a light walk if you're up to it or practice some gentle form of exercise. If you are forced to make a choice between sleeping and exercising, always choose sleep. But if you find yourself making this choice all too often, examine what needs to be changed in your life because something does.

## SMASH*N YOUR FITNESS GOALS—MOVEMENT

Movement can mean scheduled exercise or cardio workouts, but it can also mean the simple act of moving. There are many ways you can fit movement into your day, but it should be practical. Walking over to your colleague to convey information instead of sending an email is a technique that is often prescribed. Emails seem to be more about documentation than laziness anyway, and it's more efficient to dash off a message versus chit-chatting for 15 minutes over something that takes you just 1 minute. Exercising during your lunch hour is another suggestion that has legs for those who have a lunch hour to begin with or access to an exercise space, but it may be hard to fit in some movement on a street littered with obstacles like crowds, hawkers and sometimes, the street itself.

Either way, you don't have to take technology lying down. Find your own ways of squeezing movement into the day. From doing more household chores to walking short distances for errands, experiment with ways that work for you. For me, the sneakiest way to add more movement is to walk while I'm on calls. If you have calls to make—5-minute chats with your carpenter or 60-minute conference calls—talk and walk at the same time. It doesn't take any extra time, and it's a break from sitting. From struggling to finding time for movement, this one simple lifestyle change will add thousands of steps to your day. If you do this for just four to five calls of 10 minutes each, you would have walked for 40 extra minutes! Do try and walk with headphones or earphones, though. Talking for long periods with your phone held up to your ear may cause muscle imbalances, and exercises to ease them can be found in the bonus Posture Stacks at the end of Chapter 3.

You could also have the last laugh by using *technology* to bring more movement into your life. If your work requires a lot of sitting, do what I do and set phone alarms for 5 minutes each hour to get up and walk around, which will easily get you to 6000 steps over a twelve-hour day. Or use treadmills with standing desks, which are trending right now. There are also smart watches that help you monitor your movement or fitness apps that help you stick to your goals—tools that not only make you more aware of how much you've done but also potentially motivate you to do more.

Your body has a use-it-or-lose-it policy and at some point, that policy expires. The more you move, the more you *can* move. Movement doesn't require large spaces and you can make do with what you have. Whenever I get asked to speak at an event, I make the usually seated audience get up and move, which of course makes me very popular. If you're here and reading this book, chances are you have an extra 5 minutes, so why don't we get a little movement while you read? All you need is a chair:

## YASMIN'S FIVE GET-OFF-YOUR-BUTT EXERCISES

You can either follow the instructions for the exercises (listed below) or scan the QR code and select the workout to exercise with me.

What you need: A strong, secure chair (without wheels)

### MOVEMENT EXERCISE 1: CHAIR SQUAT

**What is it:** As the name suggests, you have to squat using a chair by 'pretending' to sit on it and then standing up.

**Steps:**

1. Stand in front of a chair with your back to it and your feet shoulder-width apart.
2. Bend at the hips to lower the glutes towards the chair.
3. Brush your hips to the chair and stand back up.
4. Repeat Step 3 for 1 minute.

**Check your form:** Make sure your knees don't extend over your feet, and take care to keep your back neutral and not rounded.

## MOVEMENT EXERCISE 2: TRICEPS DIPS

**What is it:** Dipping your body off the edge of a chair, using your triceps.

**Steps:**

1. Sit on a chair with your knees bent, hands next to the glutes and fingers pointing forward.
2. Extend your elbows to lift your hips off the chair so that they are hovering.
3. Bend the elbows to lower the hips down towards the floor and then extend the elbows to come back up.
4. Repeat Step 3 for 1 minute.

**Progression:** To make triceps dips more challenging, you can extend your legs further ahead at the time of getting into position.

**Check your form:**

1. Make sure your fingers are pointed in the direction of your feet.
2. While lowering your body, make sure that your knees are over your ankles.
3. Do not shrug your shoulders.
4. Bend at the elbows.
5. Keep your hips close to the chair throughout the movement.

## MOVEMENT EXERCISE 3: CHAIR PUSH-UP

**What is it:** As the name suggests, using a chair to do push-ups.

**Steps:**

1. Stand facing a chair.
2. Place your hands on the seat or on the arms of the chair, your wrist under your shoulders.
3. Straighten your legs to come into a plank with your body in a straight line from your head to your heels.
4. Bend the elbows to lower the chest towards the chair, keeping the body in a straight line.
5. Extend the elbows to come back up.
6. Repeat Steps 4 and 5 for 1 minute.

**Check your form:**

1. Make sure your body remains straight, from your head to your heels.
2. Bend at your elbows.
3. Keep your neck and spine neutral.
4. Don't forget to engage your abdominals, and squeeze your glutes.

## MOVEMENT EXERCISE 4: ALTERNATE KNEE LIFT TO CRUNCH

**What is it:** Abdominal exercises that can be done on the chair.

**Steps:**

1. Sit upright on a chair, your knees bent and feet hip-width apart. Interlace your fingers and place your hands behind your head.
2. Lift one knee towards the chest simultaneously contracting the upper body towards that knee.
3. Lower the foot and straighten the back to come back to the starting position. Repeat with the other leg.
4. Alternate legs for 1 minute.

**Check your form:**

1. Make sure your elbows are wide and not bending inwards.
2. Keep your arms behind your head.
3. Engage your abdominals.

## MOVEMENT EXERCISE 5: CHAIR JACK KNIFE

**What is it:** Abdominal exercises that can be done on the chair.

**Steps:**

1. Start by sitting on a chair. Hold the chair at the sides, behind your hips, and straighten your legs front of you.
2. Hover your feet off the floor as you lean back.
3. Contract both your upper body and your legs towards each other, bending your knees.
4. Extend both away from each other.
5. Repeat Steps 3 and 4 for 1 minute.

**Check your form:**

1. Try not to shrug your shoulders.
2. Engage your abdominals.

## SMASH*N YOUR FITNESS GOALS—ATTITUDE

I had a client. Let's call her Ragi-knee. She went for a monsoon trek and slipped on her way down a hill. She broke her fall with her knees, and she was lucky it wasn't worse. Coincidentally, she had just joined our gym and after the requisite recovery period, her physiotherapist had cleared her for exercise. But despite repeated calls and follow-ups, she was so apprehensive about restarting her sessions that she let her membership lapse with the response that she was still in a 'little pain'. While her donation to our enterprise was welcome, she didn't get much out of her time with us. The fact that to regain optimum usage of her knee, her knee had to be *used,* was not something she could be convinced about. She regained the weight she had lost, putting even more pressure on the knees she wanted to save, further relegating her to inactivity.

Every body comes with its own built-in limitations and possibilities. What you can easily do, others may not be able to. Some people have natural stamina, some are innately more muscular. Some have inborn flexibility while some have inherently weak cores. But what allows you to transcend your limitations is your attitude. So many people come in with the outlook of *'oh, my knee hurts, I can't work out'* or *'my back hurts, I can't do this.'* To them, my conversations usually go a bit like this:

Client: *Hi, Yasmin. I can't come in today. My knee hurts.*
Yasmin: Are your arms hurting?
Client: *No.*
Yasmin: Your back?
Client: *No.*
Yasmin: Your shoulders?
*Client: No.*
Yasmin: It sounds like you can do an upper body workout today. See you soon.

If your knees hurt, do an upper body workout. If your back hurts, there are exercises you can do without affecting it. If your shoulders ache, there are many lower body exercises to choose from. If your entire body hurts, do breath work like meditation, yoga or pranayama. There are as many exercises as they are excuses not to do them.

Even if your joints or muscles hurt, you can only alleviate it through *movement*. That is what physiotherapists *do*. That is what doctors *advise*. I have yet to see someone regain their fitness by doing nothing but what I have seen is that people find the quickest way to give up on something. Can't plank for more than five seconds? *'It's not for me.'* Can't do a push-up? *'I don't have upper body strength.'* Can't run on the treadmill? *'I have smoker's lungs.'*

Move to overcome the ailment you have, because if you don't, the ailment will overcome you. Of course, you need to listen to your body. Of course, you need to work out at your own pace. Of course, there will be days where you won't be able to work out at all or it could be dangerous if you attempted exercising too soon—women who want to start working out too quickly post-partum, I am talking to you—but you *must* be attuned to what your body needs, which is ultimately to move.

The same holds true for the uninjured lot who are easily dejected when they don't immediately see the results they expect. They may have been working out for weeks, desperate to make the needle move or a dress fit, but suddenly give it all up when neither happens (ignoring the other benefits like better sleep, sharper focus and mood enhancement). By trying to reverse *years* of inactivity over just a few weeks or months, you've given an ultimatum to your body without taking into consideration that your body may simply be on its own timeline. I have yet to see someone succeed with a negative attitude towards their results, but I have seen wonders being performed by those who persevered. You've tried quitting. It didn't work. How about sticking around?

## SMASH*N YOUR FITNESS GOALS—STRENGTH TRAINING

If bones are the body's framework, muscles are the plinth upon which are constructed all fitness dreams known to man. But strength training is almost always misunderstood and often ignored. To work the muscles is to build them, this is true. But, to build them is to look beefy and big, this is a misconception. To that I say, if only. If it were that easy to build muscle, people like me wouldn't have anything to do.

Like the fitness industry itself, strength training is plagued with its own set of misconceptions, and many of these are difficult to shake off. I thought I'd bust some of the greatest myths that stubbornly persist:

**Coming in at Number 3:**

# #3 The misconception that cardio burns more fat than strength training.

Perhaps you're a dedicated daily-walker. You rise with the sun and dutifully pound the pavement six days a week, but you are not seeing the results you want. Chances are you *won't*, because walking is not designed to build muscle, and it is muscle you need when you want to burn fat. The more muscle you have, the more your body burns at *rest*. This makes strength training the ultimate game changer*—you need strength *and* cardiovascular training to burn fat.

**Staying steady in the runner-up position:**

# #2 'If I stop strength training, my muscle will convert into fat.'

Fat is made of up fat cells. Muscles are made up of fibre. Fat cells cannot become fibrous any more than fibre can become fatty. The only reason muscular people look as lean as they do

---

* 'The truth behind six strength training myths,' *The University of Texas MD Anderson Cancer Center*, accessed 12 October 2022, https://www.mdanderson.org/publications/focused-on-health/thetruthbehindsixstrengthtrainingmyths.h12-1590624.html.

is because the body burns more *fat* at rest when you have more muscle. Apart from the workout your body gets while strength training, the presence of muscle boosts your metabolism hours after you've left the gym.

## Remaining undisputed at Number 1:

# #1

**Women think that weight training means that they will bulk up.**
This is the #1 reservation that most of my female clients have when they start working out—if they start building muscle, their biceps will be seen from space. To that I say that women produce more oestrogen and not as much testosterone, which is what is required for muscle building. Therefore, not only will your biceps *not* be seen from space, it will take time for them to be seen by *you*.

My niece, now an actor, had similar misgivings. When she first came to me about getting in shape, I told her that she needed to build muscle. She was all *no, no, no, I'll look too muscular*. And I was all *no, no, no, listen to your aunt*. I thought I could explain it to you the same way I explained it to her:

Number 1: If you wish to look lean and toned—that is, if you would like to have the 'celebrity' body or just look better in your clothes—you will need to train with weights. If you don't, you can exercise till the cows come home and you will still not get into *that* shape. There is no dietary or cardio substitute to getting there.

Number 2: Seeing visible muscle tone is like peeling an onion. When you first start strength training, your muscles will build faster than your fat will burn but as you continue with the weights, the fat starts to come off in layers, revealing your true muscle tone underneath. My niece, for example, took six months to see the actual shape of her shoulders and arms. It takes time, but it does happen.

Number 3: Strength training is not just about looking better in your clothes; its real purpose, as the name suggests, is to make you stronger. The older we get, the frailer we become, the frailer our bones become. You don't always have to work out with weights—simple body weight exercises can also build strength—but if you literally sit and do nothing, you allow yourself to age without fighting back. Muscle protects your bones, so when you work on them, you delay ageing and improve the quality of your life no matter when you start or how old you are.

I don't have a Number 4.

A future where we become physically weaker is already here. Strength training has the power to change or delay that outcome. However, the caveat to all good weight training programmes is to simultaneously take care of nutrition. Otherwise, you will have to wait far longer between muscle definition and fat burning, and during that interim period, you *will* start to look bulky. This period is usually when people get discouraged, stop weight training and gain even more weight. To them, I say: keep calm and keep training. You will be rewarded.

## SMASH*N YOUR FITNESS GOALS—HYDRATION

I was eating out with a friend once and she called for a cola. I asked her why. She replied saying that she didn't care for the taste of water and that a cola was '*just flavoured water, so what was the big deal, Yas? Uff!*'

Whatever I may say about the fitness industry with a capital F, I cannot deny that we have come a long way from the perception that aerated and sweetened beverages are relatively innocuous thirst quenchers and substitutes for water. We now know that they contain over ten teaspoons of sugar on an average, are loaded with difficult-to-burn empty calories, hasten tooth decay, and quench your thirst in the short-term but leave you thirstier in the medium-term. The same goes for diet drinks that contain harmful artificial sweeteners, leading to sugar cravings in the long run. It doesn't matter how much fresh fruit or veggies your diet has; you still need water.

Like sleep, hydration is a fundamental determinant of biological efficiency and dehydration adversely impacts both brain and body. It also contributes to a lack of sleep, which has a cascading effect on our fitness, as we learnt at the beginning of the chapter. You would consume a lot more water if you knew that it boosted metabolism by about 25 per cent for about an hour after you drink it.[*] If just one glass of water could do that, think of how much better your metabolism would be if you drank throughout the day. Of course, there is such a thing as *too* much water, and the ideal amount is no more than 3–4 litres a day, which you should and must consume.

Dehydration also reduces your overall strength.[†] The more dehydrated you are, the less fluid your blood will be. And the thicker the blood, the more compromised its ability to carry oxygen to your muscles. Muscles that don't get enough oxygen

---

[*] '4 Ways to Boost Your Metabolism,' *Select Health*, accessed 12 October 2022, https://selecthealth.org/blog/2018/01/4-ways-to-boostyour-metabolism.

[†] Ibid.

don't function as well, affecting your workout and ultimately your results. Severely dehydrated muscles cramp as well, which can be painful.

Consider these relatively painless ways to drink more water:

1. Drink as soon as you wake up. Your body has had no water for hours and will be thirsty.
2. Carry a bottle of water with you wherever you go, and sip when you get a chance. You can also buy water bottles that help you track your water intake, complete with markings that indicate both quantity and the time it was consumed.
3. Drink a glass of water for every hour that you are awake and stop about two hours before bedtime.* That adds up to 12–16 glasses—or the recommended 3–4 litres—a day, which is plenty.
4. If you're one of those people who don't like its taste, infuse it with flavour by adding a piece of lemon or celery or a cucumber, but *don't* juice it.
5. Don't drink water after a meal, drink it pre-meal. Drinking water during or after your meals dilutes the nutrients and their subsequent absorption by your body.
6. I often get asked about water substitutes and unfortunately, there is no such thing. That said, there are some wonderful and healthy adjuncts to it, and must be also consumed for their benefits:
   **Coconut water:** High in potassium, magnesium and phosphorus and low in calories, it has antioxidant and skin-

---

* 'Drinking Water Before Bed,' *Healthline*, accessed 12 October 2022, https://www.healthline.com/health/drinking-water-beforebed# drinking-before-bed.

friendly properties. It may even help lower blood sugar levels, boost heart health and prevent the formation of kidney stones[*].

**Buttermilk or thin** *chaas:* It is loaded with good-for-you qualities from aiding digestion to oral health, to the presence of vitamins and minerals, to being an immunity booster and helping with weight loss.[†] It's also quite filling, which makes it a great in-between snack.

**Fresh lime water:** It brings with it properties that help with skin health, digestion, immunity, heart health and lowering blood pressure. It also has anti-inflammatory and cancer-fighting benefits.[‡]

**Fresh fruits and vegetables:** In addition to their many gifts, they also have water content which helps keep you hydrated.

For best fitness results, run a mile from:

**Fruit juice:** I have lost count of the number of people I know who still think that fruit juice—freshly squeezed or packaged—is healthy. It is the opposite of healthy. Juicing strips the fruit of its fibre and changes its active ingredient to fructose, a very sugary compound. And no matter how much extra vitamins and minerals are added, packaged fruit juices are little else but sugary water.

Do remember that it takes an average of *three* oranges to make a glass of juice, but you probably won't eat more than

---

[*] '7 Science-Based Health Benefits of Coconut Water,' *Healthline*, accessed 12 October 2022, https://www.healthline.com/nutrition/coconut-water-benefits#7.-Delicious-source-of-hydration.

[†] 'Is Buttermilk Good For You,' *PharmEasy*, accessed 12 October 2022, https://pharmeasy.in/blog/health-benefits-of-buttermilk/.

[‡] '8 Benefits of Lime Water for Health and Weight Loss,' *Healthline*, accessed 12 October 2022, https://www.healthline.com/health/foodnutrition/lime-water-benefits.

one at a time. Substitute fruit juices with vegetable juices, which are far healthier.

**Aerated drinks, diet or regular:** This is one of the worst things you can do to your body and has a list of ingredients that can rival those on household cleaners. Please note that whatever you are seeing on the label is what you are putting *into* your body; and these are things that are just not meant to be there. Let us explore a label of one popular diet drink:

### Ingredients

Carbonated water, Caramel Colour, Phosphoric and Citric Acid, Aspartame (contains Phenylalanine), Flavour, Sodium Benzoate, Caffeine, Acesulfame-Potassium

I often hear that it's 'better' to have the non-diet version of colas. No, it is not better. You may be eliminating unhealthy artificial sweeteners, but you're replacing them with over ten teaspoons of sugar.* Delicious.

7. **Tea and Coffee:** Tread carefully with teas and coffees. They are not considered water and do the opposite—they dehydrate you. To prevent the acidic effects of black coffee and to make my body more alkaline, I line my stomach with

---

* 'How much sugar is actually in Coke - and what's the difference between Diet Coke and Coke Zero?' *GoodTo*, accessed 12 October 2022, https://www.goodto.com/food/sugar-in-coke-524085;(for 500 ml).

a teaspoon of coconut oil first thing in the morning before drinking my first cup of black coffee.

There was a school of thought that suggested that one shouldn't drink water while working out, which of course was later debunked. That said, sip water but don't gulp; gulping can make you feel thirstier in the long run.* If you're feeling thirsty, drink—before, during, after your workouts, it doesn't matter.

While their purpose is to replace lost electrolytes, sports drinks are recommended only if you have had an excessively taxing workout of over 60 minutes. Do bear in mind that sports drinks contain sugar that could cancel the calories burned during your workout, so they are best had after a particularly vigorous training session. If you can manage with water, nothing like it.

## SMASH*N YOUR FITNESS GOALS—NUTRITION

It is out of respect for the people who know me from the old days that I would not like to come across as some sort of fount of nutritional wisdom in these pages. Because anyone who knows me will remember me as the girl who would order not one but two chocolate mousses at a time. If my friends—at considerable risk to their lives—would dip their greedy spoons in my bowl, I would order a third mousse.

A former inhaler of dessert, an erstwhile orderer of junk and a one-time empress of third helpings, I was also someone who people assumed they could come to for nutritional advice. Only I knew how laughable that was. I knew how to counsel them, of course, because I had studied the theory, but I also knew that, if ever tested, I would fail the practical. It is only when I got my

---

* 'Chugging Water Vs. Sipping Water: Is One Better Than The Other?' *Science ABC*, accessed 12 October 2022, https://www.scienceabc.com/humans/chugging-water-vs-sipping-water-one-better.html.

own act together that I began to see results I hadn't seen in my twenties and thirties.

The belief that if you exercise, you can eat whatever you want, is unfortunately just a myth and *'you can't out-exercise a bad diet.'*I can give you all the exercise programmes in the universe, but statistically only 25–30% of weight loss is due to exercise, which means that the balance 70–75% depends heavily on what you eat. These are, of course, broad numbers, but the fact remains that the roles of nutrition and lifestyle combined are more important than exercise in fitness. Note that I didn't use the word 'diet' but the word 'nutrition', and the reason I do that is because diets are not always sustainable, but nutrition is.

People are born with different fat-to-muscle ratios and varying degrees of metabolic efficiency, which is why the food plans that work for your friend may not suit you. That said, there are some things that all good nutritional approaches have in common. While I am not a nutrition expert, I can share what my eating principles are, in the hope that these may inspire you to craft a plan for your own unique body type. These are not based on any fad or trend, but are part trial-and-error and mostly good, old-fashioned common sense:

1.  **I try to be a food snob** by prioritizing ingredients that are *quality-dense*. For example, almonds are high in calories, but they are a wonderful source of fibre, healthy fats and energy. Avocados are high in fat but rich in folates, potassium, good fats and fibre. Other quality foods include broccoli, eggs, milk, quinoa, onions, spinach and other leafy greens, dals, carrots, fruit, lean meats and paneer. Even a casual search on nutrient-dense, quality foods will reveal options that fit your

'6 Reasons Why You Can't Out-Exercise a Bad Diet,' *Daily Burn*, accessed 8 December 2022, https://dailyburn.com/life/health/exercise-weight-loss-diet/.

palate, lifestyle and budget, and you'd be surprised to find that the best superfoods have been chilling in your fridge all along.

Fast food, aerated drinks, sugary desserts, many fried foods, and packaged or processed foods are *quality-poor* and I avoid them as much as possible. Bereft of nutritional benefit, refried in toxic oils or teeming with chemicals that are not meant to be part of the thriving ecosystem in our bodies, these foods are called junk for a reason. Do with these foods what you do with garbage and throw them away.

2.  **I try to eat home-cooked food.** Commercially prepared foods are designed with repeat purchase in mind and consequently, most are loaded with sugar and fat. To make the business of food profitable, many also contain cheaper substitutes and low-quality oils that inflame your insides. That said, if I completely ban eating out or eating packaged foods, I wouldn't have either friends or family, but I try to keep it to a minimum because I don't want to die alone.

3.  **I try to differentiate between need and greed.** At what point does need stop and greed start? Hunger is only *one* of the reasons we eat—there's social eating, eating for greed, eating for comfort, eating for taste. Our hunger levels also fluctuate on a daily basis—on some days we are hungrier, other days not so much. Understanding the difference between what my eyes want and what my body needs has been a lesson that has taken me a lifetime to perfect, but I promise you it's an enterprise worth embarking on. Eyes can be closed.

4.  **I try and choose foods that prioritize gut health.** The gut is our body's largest digestive organ and while its importance has been underscored in ancient texts for millennia, it is only now being identified as one of the biggest determinants of our well-being. The walls of our intestine have something called villi—small projections that absorb nutrients and water—that send these nutrients throughout your body. However and unfortunately, the same applies for toxins.

May you never have to see the inside of a sewer pipe, but if you do, you may observe years of waste deposited on the inside walls. In the same way, leftover waste and toxins from undigested food can deposit on the inner walls of your intestines and stay there for years. The villi will absorb these toxins and dispatch them to different parts of your body. If they reach your skin, you may get pimples. If they reach your kidneys, you may get kidney stones. Most detox programmes are really gut cleanses with the objective of restoring gut health so that your body is better able to absorb nutrients. There are also some gut-healthy foods you can try to include:

1. Chewing ginger with black salt
2. Ash gourd
3. Coconut
4. Buttermilk infused with cumin, curry leaves and ginger
5. Kashaya tea (prepared with coriander seeds, cumin seeds and fennel seeds)
6. Black raisins
7. Khichdi
8. Kodo millet
9. Black carrot kanji
10. Beetroot kanji
11. Gond katira
12. Turmeric
13. Ghee rice
14. Methi kanji

And along with the food, try these tips to maintain or restore gut health:

1. Be relaxed and comfortable while eating.
2. Listen to your body and know when to stop eating.
3. Eat good quality food at warm temperatures.
4. Focus on your meal.
5. Eat food at a reasonable time.
6. Don't forget to chew!

5. **I try to eat balanced meals.** As much as possible, I make it point to balance my plate with good sources of protein, good fats, complex carbohydrates and fibre. These not only help me fuel my workouts, but also significantly reduce my cravings.

6. **I try and eat as per my circadian rhythm.** Defined in terms of twenty-four-hour cycles, a circadian rhythm is the clock your body follows from morning to night. Whether we're late-sleepers or early-risers, we each have our own body clock. We may not always consciously be aware of it, but we have an assigned time for most of our activities, from bathing to working out to getting ready for bed. Ever felt tired, weak, irritable, constipated or unwell from an erratic schedule? That's your body complaining that you're doing things it can't process. I try to eat as per my body clock and get my last meal in at least three hours before bedtime.

7. **I never test fads on my body.** Extreme dieting was never my thing, even when I was at my unhealthiest. I'd advise you to never follow a diet that excludes a whole food group like carbohydrates or fats. Carbohydrates mentally satisfy you and also help relieve stress if eaten in the right proportion. That's why carbohydrate-laden foods are often comfort food. The same goes for fats—your body needs a certain proportion for basic functioning that you should never go without.

8. **I never starve.** Starvation is the *worst* thing you can do to your body, and it includes skipping meals because you're compensating for an eating binge. Apart from interfering with your body's functioning, you will lose muscle over time if you consistently starve. And if you lose muscle, do remember what we discussed in the first chapter— fat occupies the space that muscle leaves. You will gain nothing from starvation except weight.

## YASMIN'S TRIED-AND-TESTED PRE-WORKOUT SNACKS:

1. **Bananas with Nuts**
2. **Yoghurt with Fruit**
3. **Apple Wedges with Peanut Butter**
4. **Homemade Seed Bars**

5. **Grain-Free Seed Crackers**

*What you need:*

1. ⅓ cup sunflower seeds
2. ⅓ cup pumpkin seeds
3. ⅓ cup chia seeds
4. 1 cup flaxseeds
5. ⅓ cup sesame seeds
6. Dry seasoning of your choice
7. ½ teaspoon oregano
8. 1 teaspoon garlic powder
9. ½ teaspoon chilli flakes
10. ¾ teaspoon rock salt
11. 300 ml water

*Method:*

1. Mix all the seeds in a bowl.
2. Add seasoning and water and mix well.
3. Cover the bowl and refrigerate for four to five hours. The chia seeds will absorb the water and develop a jelly-like consistency.
4. Pre-heat the oven for 10 minutes at 120°C.
5. Spread the mixture thinly on a baking sheet and bake for 1½ hours until crisp.

6.  Your crackers are ready!
7.  You can also pair it with this easy-to-make hung curd dip—
    hang some curd in a cheesecloth for about an hour, and to
    that add crushed garlic, salt, pepper and chilli flakes.

## 6. Rice Cake Crispy Bars*

*This vegan, gluten-free, four-ingredient recipe is designed to
cover all your chocolate cravings.*

*For the bars:*

1.  8 rice cakes
2.  80 grams dairy-free chocolate, melted
3.  2 tablespoons peanut butter
4.  ¼ cup vegan chocolate protein powder

*For the topping:*

1.  40 grams dark chocolate, melted
2.  1 tablespoon peanut butter
3.  1 teaspoon maple syrup
4.  1 tablespoon vegan chocolate protein powder

*Method:*

1.  In a bowl, add the melted dairy-free chocolate, peanut butter
    and protein powder and mix until smooth.
2.  In another bowl, crumble the rice cakes into small chunks.
3.  Pour the mixture of the first bowl on to the crumbled rice
    cakes and fold until the cakes are fully coated by the mixture.
4.  Transfer into a container or on to a small baking tray lined
    with non-stick paper and press down until flat and even.

---

* Recipe inspired from: https://www.instagram.com/reel/CefpEobIgha/?
  igshid=YmMyMTA2M2Y=

5. In a separate bowl, make the topping by mixing the melted chocolate, maple syrup, peanut butter and protein powder together, and pour over the coated rice cakes.
6. Pop the rice cakes in the freezer to set for 30 minutes before slicing.

**7. Mango Sabja Pudding**

*What you need:*

1. 1 mango
2. 1 tablespoon sabja (sweet basil) seeds
3. 1 teaspoon maple syrup
4. ½ cup of coconut milk
5. Few drops of vanilla essence

*Method:*

1. In a bowl, add the sabja seeds, maple syrup, vanilla essence and coconut milk and mix until the seeds are fully immersed.
2. Keep the mixture aside for 5–10 minutes until the seeds swell and absorb the liquid.
3. Cut the mango into small cubes.
4. In a glass, alternately layer the mango cubes with the sabja mixture.
5. Top off with chunks of mango, and sprinkle with chopped nuts, if you like.

**8. Nutty Stuffed Dates**

*What you need:*

1. 12 Medjool dates
2. ⅓ cup smooth peanut butter

3.  ¼ cup peanuts, crushed
4.  ½ cup semi-sweet chocolate chips
5.  A pinch of sea salt (optional)

*Method:*

1.  Slice each date lengthwise, and remove the pit.
2.  Stuff each date with peanut butter and sprinkle it with the crushed peanuts.
3.  Drizzle the melted chocolate chips over the dates to coat.
4.  You can also sprinkle sea salt, if you like.
5.  Refrigerate the stuffed dates until the chocolate has fully hardened.

## YASMIN'S TRIED-AND-TESTED POST-WORKOUT SNACKS:

1.  **Vegetable Omelette with Avocado**
2.  **Avocado on Gluten-Free or Sourdough Bread**
3.  **Peanut Butter and Half a Banana**
4.  **Chia Pudding**
5.  **Oats Porridge (100 grams) with Any One Fruit, along with A Handful of Nuts**
6.  **Hummus and Carrot Sticks**

7.  **Cinnamon Protein Balls**

*For the balls:*

1.  ¼ cup protein powder
2.  ½ cup almond butter
3.  3 tablespoons desiccated coconut flour
4.  2 tablespoons maple syrup
5.  1 tablespoon cinnamon

*For the coating:*

1.  1 tablespoon cinnamon
2.  2 tablespoons desiccated coconut flour

*Method:*

1.  In a bowl, add all the ingredients for the balls and mix to make a dough.
2.  Roll the dough into balls.
3.  For the coating, mix the cinnamon and coconut flour.
4.  Roll each ball into the mixture and refrigerate it for 10 minutes.

## 8.  Chocolate Peanut Butter Pops*

*For the bars:*

1.  2 ripe bananas
2.  ¼ cup peanut butter
3.  1 cup almond milk
4.  ½ cup protein powder of your choice (you can substitute protein powder by adding more bananas and using less almond milk)

*For the topping:*

1.  ⅓ cup melted dark chocolate (I use 85 per cent dark chocolate, but it is up to you)
2.  2 tablespoons peanuts

---

* Recipe inspired by: https://www.instagram.com/reel/Cd5n_sdAGwM/?igshid=YmMyMTA2M2Y%3D

*Method:*

1.  In a bowl, smash the bananas using a fork, then add peanut butter, protein powder and milk and mix well until you get a creamy texture.
2.  Pour the mixture into popsicle moulds and freeze for 5 to 6 hours.
3.  For the topping, mix the melted dark chocolate with the peanuts, and dip each frozen popsicle into the mixture.
4.  A tip: if the chocolate is slightly warm, it will freeze over the cold popsicle immediately! You can additionally sprinkle some crushed peanuts on it to further enhance the taste.

### 9.  Yummy Healthy Chocolate Bites

*What you need (quantities of your choice):*

1.  Bananas
2.  Strawberries
3.  Green apples
4.  Peanut butter
5.  Dark chocolate

*Method:*

1.  Slice the fruits.
2.  Take two slices of the same fruit and make a sandwich with a layer of peanut butter in between. Freeze for an hour.
3.  Melt dark chocolate of your liking and coat the fruit sandwich with it.
4.  Freeze until the chocolate solidifies.

## 10. Post-workout Balls*

*What you need:*

1. 120 grams red dates
2. 30 grams/2 tablespoons semi-crushed almonds
3. 2 tablespoons almond oil
4. 2 tablespoons desiccated coconut
5. ¼ teaspoon cinnamon
6. ½ teaspoon elaichi powder
7. 2 tablespoons cocoa powder
8. 2 tablespoons chia seeds powder
9. 2 tablespoons alsi/flaxseed powder
10. 2 tablespoons black raisins
11. 1 tablespoon fresh grated ginger/ginger candy
12. 2 tablespoons pumpkin seeds, crushed or powdered
13. 2 tablespoons sunflower seeds, crushed or powdered

*Method:*

1. Crush the dates in a mixer.
2. Add all the above ingredients.
3. Mix it thoroughly.
4. Make small balls (lemon size).

# YASMIN'S TRIED-AND-TESTED ANYTIME GO-TO RECIPES:

## 1. Yasmin's Go-To Cappuccino

*What you need:*

1. 1 cup hot water

---

* Recipe Credit: Shweta Shah, Eatfit 24/7

2.  1½ teaspoons coffee
3.  1 teaspoon coconut sugar
4.  ¼ cup coconut milk/milk of your choice
5.  Cinnamon powder to garnish

*Method:*

1.  Add the water, coffee, sugar and milk to a blender and blend.
2.  Pour into a cup and top off with cinnamon powder to taste.

**2.  Rainbow Salad**

*For the dressing:*

1.  ¼ teaspoon orange zest
2.  2 tablespoons orange juice, freshly squeezed
3.  ½ teaspoon apple cider vinegar or lemon juice
4.  ¼ teaspoon olive oil
5.  2 teaspoons fresh oregano leaves
6.  Salt and pepper to taste

*For the salad:*

1.  ½ cup mixed bell peppers, chopped into cubes
2.  ¼ cup blanched broccoli
3.  2 tablespoons shredded carrot
4.  2 tablespoons onion, chopped

*Method:*

1.  Mix all the ingredients for the dressing and refrigerate.
2.  Just before you're ready to eat, combine all the salad ingredients in a salad bowl, add the dressing and toss well.
3.  Serve cold.

### 3.   Rich Dark Chocolate Granola

*What you need:*

1.  4 cups rolled oats
2.  ½ cup mixed berries
3.  ⅓ cup 100 per cent cocoa powder
4.  ½ cup sunflower seeds
5.  ½ cup pecans
6.  1 tablespoon cinnamon
7.  ½ teaspoon Himalayan salt
8.  ½ cup maple syrup
9.  ½ cup coconut oil
10. 2 teaspoons vanilla extract

*Method:*

1.  To a baking tray, add the oats, mixed berries, cocoa powder, sunflower seeds, pecans, cinnamon and Himalayan salt and mix well.
2.  To this, add maple syrup, coconut oil and the vanilla extract, and mix well.
3.  Preheat your oven to 180°C and bake for 30 minutes.

### 4.   Watermelon Cooler*

*What you need:*

1.  1 watermelon (half will be used)
2.  2 tablespoons mint leaves
3.  ½ teaspoon rock salt

---

* Recipe inspired by: https://www.instagram.com/reel/CbXc2KhtuxD/?igshid=YmMyMTA2M2Y%3D

4. Jeera powder
5. Juice of half a lemon

*Method:*

1. Cut a watermelon in half.
2. Take one watermelon half, scoop out six to eight balls of watermelon and keep them aside.
3. Scoop out the leftover watermelon, transfer it to a blender and add mint leaves, rock salt, jeera powder and lemon juice and blend.
4. Strain the mixture and pour it back into the watermelon shell.
5. Now, add the watermelon balls and mint leaves.
6. Freeze and enjoy!

## 5. Rice Methi (Fenugreek) Porridge

*What you need:*

1. 2 tablespoons methi (fenugreek) seeds
2. ¼ cup rice
3. ¼ cup shredded coconut
4. 2 tablespoons jaggery
5. 1½ teaspoons cumin seeds
6. Salt to taste

*Method:*

1. Soak the methi and cumin seeds overnight. Discard the water in the morning.
2. In a pressure cooker, add the rice, shredded coconut, as well as the soaked fenugreek and cumin seeds with two cups of water and salt to taste.

3. Cook for two whistles or until it is done. Open the lid, and add the jaggery.
4. Transfer into a bowl, garnish with 1 teaspoon of ghee and serve hot.

*

## How much protein does your body need?

I see much fuss being made about the relationship between protein and fitness, so I thought it could be addressed here. For the purposes of protein consumption, I've divided the world into two kinds of people—those who want to be fit (Population A) and those who want to gain muscle (Population B).

Population A: For those who want be healthy, toned and fit, your daily intake of protein should be enough so long as you're having good quality protein for breakfast, lunch and dinner, which includes sprouts, poha, oatmeal with a variety of nuts and seeds, nut or seed butter, paneer, eggs, alfalfa sprouts, sattu, chicken, fish and dahi.

Population B: If a significant amount of muscle gain is your goal, I still believe you can attain it by eating good quality protein. But if you are not seeing results, use protein supplements that are anti-inflammatory, natural and that don't include sugars or sweeteners—like sucralose, maltodextrin and dextrose—which could imbalance the gut microbiome. Do bear in mind that many commercially available protein supplements are hard to digest and excess consumption may cause gas and bloating. If you find that this is not working for you, drop the supplements and get your protein needs solely from food.

*

Over the course of my career, I have found that while the clients change, the questions remain the same. They all come in with an expectation of a number that they had in mind for weight loss. They would tell me that they wanted to lose five kilos in three months, for example, but my response was always the same: I have absolutely *no* idea how much you will lose. I lost a lot of clients early on with this approach, and even if you come to me now and ask me the same question, I still won't be able to give you an answer after thirty years in the business, because each body is different, and each person reacts differently to the same programme. I train the body I see in front of me.

What we weigh can never be solely attributed to the accumulation of fat—water content, bone density or muscle mass all have a role to play. If we judge ourselves only by a number on a scale, we are ignoring other equally important parameters like how well our clothes fit, how we feel and how much more energy we have. Muscle weighs more than fat and especially early on in your fitness journey, you may temporarily weigh more after an initial phase of strength training.

Predicting a weight loss target is like studying for an exam and expecting an exact grade—you may get an examiner who has their own way of assessing your effort. Replace the examiner with your body, and you'll find it does its own assessment. Fitness is the *outcome*, the result of all your hard work that you have put in thus far. That said, there *is* a magic formula to getting the body you've always wanted. And that formula is consistency. The best thing you can do for yourself is to just show up.

# PART TWO: THE WORKOUTS

*Chapter Three: Yasmin Karachiwala's*
*10-Minute Workout Stacks*
*Bonus Workouts: Posture Stacks*

# Working It Out

## *Before you start*

## *A brief guide before we start the workouts to include the QR code system and what you need before you start*

It takes a dedicated optimist to find silver linings in the COVID-19 pandemic, but I specialize in such treasure hunts because it keeps me sane. Lockdowns not only made people become far more conscious of their physical activity or lack thereof, but many also changed the way they looked at exercise—from a necessary evil to a pleasurable escape. Never have I received so many calls from people who missed working out as much as I did when the option was no longer open to them. Necessary government curbs also meant that people became more seasoned with exercising at home—and saw results—which meant that perceptions of workouts became more flexible. The exercises listed here travel well and can be done anywhere, from homes to beaches to hotel rooms to terraces. All they need is some basic equipment and, of course, you.

### Ten before you Ten

Before you embark on the exercises, here are ten things you need to keep in mind before you start:

1. Check with your **doctor** before starting any exercise programme.

2. Before you begin each workout, try and keep these **ready**—a *chair*, if the exercise calls for it (make sure your chair is secure, strong and without wheels). An *exercise mat* for stretches and floor exercises. A small *towel* or napkin. A bottle of *water*. Lastly, give yourself *enough room* to move your arms and legs.

3. You can include light **dumbbells**—or strap-on weights on your arms—to make an exercise more challenging. If you don't have dumbbells, fill two bottles of the same size with water.

4. **All exercises in this section are for a duration of 45 seconds with a 15-second break. And, as mentioned in the beginning of the book, *all* exercises are accompanied by my video instruction, which you can access by scanning the QR code and selecting the relevant exercise stack.** If your phone isn't working or Internet access is limited, the written version for each exercise **is a back-up.** If you're feeling unsure or intimidated, use **the modified version** of each exercise, where indicated. There's nothing in here that should make you feel either, but you know your body best. Alternatively, if you find the modified version challenging, start with 20 seconds, and build up to 45 seconds at your own pace.

5. At any point, if you experience **dizziness, nausea, chest pain**, or are so **breathless** that you cannot talk, that's your body telling you to stop. Please stop. With the exception of chest pain, you can resume when you stop feeling dizzy, nauseous or breathless. Chest pain needs a call to a doctor.

6. If you're doing it right, you will **not** feel knee **pain**, neck strain, lower back pain or unwelcome pain of any kind. If you feel a twinge, practice the modified version and build your strength till the twinge is gone.

7. Try **not** to eat a **heavy meal** right before your workout. Keep a gap of at least one and a half hours after major meals. If you're exercising first thing in the morning, go back to *SMASH\*N* for some pre-workout meal ideas.

8. **Take your time**. Do your exercises carefully by being present and in the moment. Distractions lead to injury.

9. **Consistency is key**. Show up six days a week. Everyone may not have a daily hour for exercise, but there is no one who doesn't have ten minutes.

10. If you are doing three or more 10-minute stacks *at a time*, you will need to **warm-up and cool-down**. I have provided some warm-up and cool-down stacks within the chapter, along with an explanation about why they are important.

Let's ten!

3

# Yasmin Karachiwala's 10-Minute Workout Stacks

## *Ready, steady, FIT*

All prescribed exercises in this chapter will be in units of ten-minute sessions and are stackable, which means that they can be done by themselves or combined with other 10-minute workouts depending on how much time you have. The only rule is that if you are doing more than one 10-minute workout in the day, it can't be the same stack. You must combine it with another stack for true benefit.

### One Stack = **10**-minute exercise session

### PICKING STACKS

Detailed in this chapter are a wide variety of stacks from lower body to cardio workouts, and have been culled from multiple disciplines to include Pilates as well as strength, functional and cardiovascular training. The stacks are no more than 10 minutes long and the first exercise of each stack warms you up for that particular stack. These exercises have been prescribed for years and some of them are favourites of the celebrities I train, and I hope you enjoy them.

You can pick stacks from the 10-Minute Stack Menu on page 77. Each stack has a target area or objective—upper body, lower body, abdominals, full body, cardio—and you can pick those that suit your objective. However, if you don't have an objective in mind, you could also follow this baseline plan for picking a stack:

1. If you have only 10 minutes, do a full-body stack, because it targets all your body parts.
2. If you feel like you've been sitting all day, and are feeling restless, do a cardio stack to get your heart pumping.
3. You can also mix it up like this:

- Monday **10-minute** full body stack
- Tuesday **10-minute** lower body stack
- Wednesday **10-minute** upper body stack
- Thursday **10-minute** abdominal stack
- Friday **10-minute** cardio stack
- Saturday **10-minute** full body stack
- Sunday **Rest**

If you do suddenly find yourself with more than 10 minutes on a Tuesday, for example, do any of the stacks mixed with cardio; it's a great combination. Or if you want to do 50 minutes, do one of each; in this way you would have covered the full body. If you only want to focus on the legs, then do four lower body workouts. You get the idea. There are no rules, but this would be a good way to start.

These workouts can be combined with a walk or a swim or any other form of exercise, but if you do have one very vigorous hour of exercise planned (other than a stack), I recommend you do no more than *one* 10-minute session for that day. If you haven't worked out in a while, I recommend picking from the modified version of the stack. Once you do these and you feel more confident, you can graduate to the more advanced version and add more stacks.

# WARM-UP AND COOL-DOWN

## Warming Up

*For three or more stacks at a time*

There is no faster way to find yourself in the company of an ice pack or a doctor than if you seek the path of skipping your warm-up. I've often felt that people don't give this crucial part of exercising the respect it deserves, and I've had to caution so many chronic latecomers to my 60-minute group classes about the consequences of either missing part of this process or just going through the motions, with the belief that the little bit they do will suffice.

It is important to warm-up with the same focus as you work out. This is because—and let me use a digital example—your body has to go from offline to online. Here it is, politely minding its business, when you decide to encase it in stretchy clothes and subject it to kicks, jumps, sweat and resistance. A warm-up is a way to *invite* your body to the journey of exercise and allow it to cooperate with your intention. Here is what happens when you warm up.[*]

*It prepares your body for what lies ahead.* A warm-up sends a signal to key organs like the heart and lungs as well as to your muscles that more of their involvement is needed, allowing your body to gently adapt to—rather than being shocked into—more strenuous activity.

*It raises the temperature of your blood.* Higher blood temperature weakens the bond between oxygen and haemoglobin.

---

[*] 'Should You Warm Up Before Exercise?' *VeryWell Fit*, accessed on 19 March 2022, https://www.verywellfit.com/how-to-warm-up-before-exercise-3119266.

This allows your body to send more blood to the parts that need it, like your muscles, and this, in turn, boosts your endurance.

*It dilates blood vessels.* A warm-up increases the flow of blood and reduces the pressure on your heart.

*It produces exercise-friendly hormones like cortisol and epinephrine.* These hormones enable your body to make more carbohydrates and fats available for energy production, leading to a better burn of what you ate.

*It gradually increases muscle temperature.* 'Warm' muscles work better than 'cold' muscles, because cold muscles are stiffer.

*It facilitates a better range of motion.* Touch your toes when your body is not warmed up and do it when it is, and you will see how much more reach you get. The better your range of motion, the more benefit your body gets from your workout.

*It provides a psychological advantage.* The process of shutting out distractions and focusing on yourself starts with the warm-up.

## Warm-up

*While this is for those attempting three stacks or more, you can also use this warm-up before embarking on any other exercise. You can either follow the steps below, or scan the QR code below to warm-up with me.*

### 1.   FRONT LEG SWINGS

1.   Stand upright with your feet hip-width apart.

2. Lift one leg off the floor and raise it as high as you can with control.

3. Bring the leg back down to touch the floor and raise again for 30 seconds.

4. Repeat on the other leg for 30 seconds.

## 2. SIDE LEG SWINGS

1. Stand upright with your feet hip-width apart.

2. Lift one leg to the side as high as you can without moving the whole body and bring it back down with control. Repeat for 30 seconds.

3. Repeat on the other leg for 30 seconds.

## 3. BACK LEG SWINGS

1. Stand upright with your feet hip-width apart.

2. Lift one leg to raise it behind you without arching your lower back.

3. Bring it back to the starting position, and repeat for 30 seconds.

4. Change legs and repeat for 30 seconds.

## 4. SHOULDER CIRCLES FORWARD

1. Stand upright with your feet hip-width apart.

2. Lift your arms out laterally to the sides at shoulder-height.

3. In this position, circle your shoulders clockwise for 30 seconds.

## 5. FRONT ARM CIRCLES

1. Stand upright with your feet hip-width apart and your arms by your sides.

2.  Lift your arms forward, then up to the ceiling, then take them behind you and come back to the starting position.
3.  Repeat for 30 seconds.

### 6.  SHOULDER CIRCLES BACK

1.  Stand upright with your feet hip-width apart.
2.  Lift your arms out laterally to the sides at shoulder-height.
3.  In this position, circle your shoulders anti-clockwise for 30 seconds.

### 7.  BACK ARM CIRCLES

1.  Stand upright with your feet hip-width apart and your arms by your sides.
2.  Lift your arms behind you, then up towards the ceiling, then bring them forward and then back down to your sides.
3.  Repeat for 30 seconds.

### 8.  HIP CIRCLES AND REVERSE

1.  Stand upright with your feet hip-width apart and your hands on your hips.
2.  Circle the hips clockwise for 15 seconds and then anti-clockwise for 15 seconds.

### 9.  SIDE BEND

1.  Stand with your feet wide, toes turned out.
2.  Lift the right arm first laterally sideways and then up towards the ceiling.
3.  Bend and flex the spine to the left.
4.  Come back to the centre and repeat on the other side.
5.  Alternate sides for a total of 1 minute.

## 10.  SIDE BEND WITH LUNGE

1.   Stand upright with your feet in a wide turned-out position.
2.   Bend your right knee, simultaneously raise your left arm and side bend your torso to the right.
3.   Come back to the centre and repeat on the other side.
4.   Alternate sides for a total of 1 minute.

## 11.  SIDE BEND WITH ROTATION

1.   Stand upright with your feet shoulder-width apart, with both arms straight up towards the ceiling and the palms facing each other like you are holding an imaginary ball.
2.   Side bend to the right. From this position, contract your torso towards the floor and come up into a side bend at the left and back to the starting position.
3.   Repeat four times on each side.

## 12.  ROLL DOWN TO PLANK

1.   Stand upright with your feet hip-width apart and your arms by your sides.
2.   Lift the arms laterally up towards the ceiling.
3.   Leading with your head, roll the spine down towards the floor, one vertebra at a time.
4.   Place your hands on the floor and 'walk' into a plank making sure that your body is in a straight line from your head to your heels.
5.   'Walk' the hands back to the feet and roll the spine back up to the starting position.
6.   Repeat for 1 minute.

You're all warmed up for your workout.

## Cooling Down

*For three or more stacks at a time*

An oft underestimated component of a workout, the 'cool-down' is usually the last 5 or 10 minutes of a session and is *not* the time to get up, grab your towel and head to the changing room.

During your workout, as your muscles get to work, there is a build-up of lactic acid in your body. This lactic acid needs to be drained—which is what a good cool-down session will do—else you will be sore or develop cramps, neither of which is useful for the rest of your day. Cool-downs also help bring your elevated heart rate back to normal.

A standard session includes stretches and a general slowing down of exercise activity. Being the conceptual opposite of warm-ups—warm ups are dynamic and you can't hold a position for too long because your muscles are still cold—you can hold a static position or a stretch for much longer during a cool-down session. This part of the workout also feels immensely rewarding, so do take advantage of it when you can.

## Cool-Down

You can either follow the steps below, or scan the QR code to cool-down with me.

### 1.  QUAD LUNGE STRETCH

1.  Start by kneeling on a mat. Bring one leg forward and straighten the back leg to come into a low lunge position. Place your hands on either side of the front foot.
2.  You can either hold this position or pulse the hip towards the floor for 30 seconds to feel the stretch in the quadriceps.

## 2.  PSOAS STRETCH

1.  From the above position, lower the back knee on the floor, and bring your torso upright.
2.  Press the hips forward to stretch the psoas or the hip flexor muscle.
3.  Hold this stretch for 30 seconds.

## 3.  HAMSTRING STRETCH

1.  From the above position, sit back on the back heel and straighten the front leg.
2.  Flex the heel of the front foot towards the ceiling to feel the stretch in the hamstring.
3.  Hold the stretch for 30 seconds.

## 4.  GLUTE STRETCH

1.  From the above position, bend the front leg in a figure 4 position, wherein the calf is on the mat, and parallel to the chest. Your forearms should be on either side, and the back leg should be straight.
2.  Lower the hip to feel the stretch in the glute.
3.  Hold the stretch for 30 seconds.

## 5.  ADDUCTOR SIDE BEND RIGHT

1.  Sit upright on a mat and open both legs as wide apart as they can go.
2.  Laterally flex the spine to do a side-bend to the right, bringing the left hand overhead.
3.  Hold this position for 30 seconds.

## 6. ADDUCTOR SIDE BEND LEFT

1. Now, laterally flex the spine to do a side-bend to the left, bringing the right hand overhead.
2. Hold this position for 30 seconds.

*Now, repeat exercises 4, 3, 2 and 1 (in that order) from the previous pages on the other side.*

## 7. CAT AND COW

1. Start in an all-fours position with your hands under your shoulders and knees under your hips.
2. Round the back from the tail to the head, flexing the spine. Then, reverse the movement by opening the back to come into an extension of the back from the tail to the top of the head.
3. Repeat Step 2 four times.

## 8. PIKE HEEL RAISES

1. From the all-fours position, take your hips up towards the ceiling, bringing the chest towards the thighs and ears, and in line with your arms to come into a pike position.
2. Bend one knee and lift the heel of the leg, pressing the other heel into the mat.
3. Alternate heel raises for 30 seconds.

## 9. SHOULDER STRETCH RIGHT

1. Stand upright and take your right arm across the chest towards the left arm, and gently pull with the left hand to stretch the shoulder.
2. Hold for 15 seconds.

## 10. TRICEPS STRETCH RIGHT

1. Take the right hand up towards the ceiling, then bend the elbow behind your head, getting the upper arm in line with the ear. Take the left hand and pull the right elbow back to stretch the triceps, and hold for 15 seconds.

## 11. SHOULDER STRETCH LEFT

1. Stand upright and take your left arm across the chest towards the right arm, and gently pull with the right hand to stretch the shoulder.
2. Hold for 15 seconds.

## 12. TRICEPS STRETCH LEFT

1. Take the left hand up towards the ceiling, then bend the elbow behind your head, getting the upper arm in line with the ear. Take the right hand and pull the left elbow back to stretch the triceps, and hold for 15 seconds.

## 13. HIP CIRCLES AND REVERSE

1. Stand upright with your feet shoulder-width apart and toes pointed out, hands on your waist.
2. Circle the hips clockwise for four counts and then anti-clockwise for four counts.

## 14. NECK STRETCH

1. Stand upright with your feet together, hands by your sides, palms facing back.
2. Press your arms back from your shoulders, opening the chest. Look to the right, and then to the left and then release the arms.

3.  Press your arms back from your shoulders, opening the chest. Look to the left, and then to the right and then release the arms.

## 15. *PLIÉ* CONTRACT AND HIGH RELEASE

1.  Stand upright with your feet together and arms by your side.
2.  Bend at the ankles to come into a *plié* simultaneously contracting the back and taking the arms forward as if you are hugging someone.
3.  Straighten your knees to stand upright, and extend your upper back to go into a high release, opening your arms up into a V.
4.  Repeat Steps 2 and 3 four times.

## 16. *RELEVÉ* WITH ARM LIFTS

1.  Stand upright with your feet together and arms by your sides.
2.  Engage the abdominals to lift the heels coming on to the balls of your feet and take the arms towards the ceiling. Lower the heels and arms back to the starting position.
3.  Repeat Step 2 for 30 seconds.

# 10-Minute Workout Stacks

# 10-Minute Stack Menu

## Upper Body Stack 3

## Upper Body Stack 4

## Upper Body Stack 5

## 10-Minute Lower Body Stacks

## Lower Body Stack 4

## Lower Body Stack 5

## 10-Minute Abdominal Stacks                               143

## Abdominal Stack 1

## Abdominal Stack 4

## Abdominal Stack 5

## 10-Minute Cardio Stacks

## Cardio Stack 1

## Full Body Stack 2

## Full Body Stack 3

## Full Body Stack 4

# 10-Minute Upper Body Stacks

## UPPER BODY STACK 1

Upper Body Stack 1 has five exercises. Each exercise will be done for 45 seconds with a 15-second break. Repeat once more to complete the 10-minute stack. You can either follow the steps below or use your phone to scan the QR code, and select  Upper Body Stack 1 from the menu to work out along with me.

### 1. INCHWORM

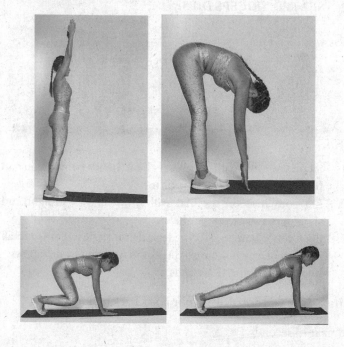

1. Stand upright with your feet hip-width apart.
2. Inhale and move your arms up.
3. Exhale and roll down towards the floor, keeping your knees as straight as possible.
4. From this position, bend your knees and 'walk' forward with your hands into a plank. Make sure that your shoulders are over your wrist and that your body is in a straight line from your head to your heels. Engage your abdominals and squeeze your glutes.
5. Bend your knees, and 'walk' back towards your feet.
6. Roll back up.
7. Repeat Steps 1 to 6 for 45 seconds.

Break: 15 seconds.

## 2. SEATED TRICEPS DIPS

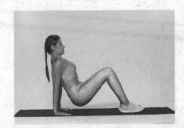
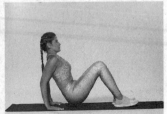

1. Sit on your mat with your knees bent, hands behind you and fingers pointing towards your toes.
2. Lift your hips off the mat with your elbows straight and shoulders away from your ears.
3. Bend your elbows and then extend them. This exercise is a small movement: you just have to bend and straighten your elbows.
4. Repeat Step 3 for 45 seconds.

**Make sure you don't sway your body back and forth.**

Break: 15 seconds.

### 3. KNEE PUSH-UPS

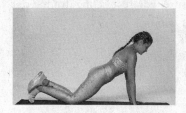 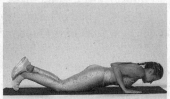

1. Kneel on the mat.
2. From this position, 'walk' out with your hands to get into a modified plank with your shoulders over your wrists and knees still on the mat. Make sure your body is in a straight line from your knees to your head. Engage your abdominals and squeeze your glutes.
3. From this position, bend your elbows to lower yourself towards the mat, and extend to push yourself back up.
4. Repeat Step 3 for 45 seconds.

Break: 15 seconds.

### 4. SHOULDER CIRCLES

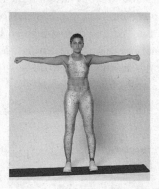

1. Stand upright with your feet hip-width apart.
2. Extend your arms out by your sides in a T.

3. Circle your shoulders in any one direction—clockwise or anticlockwise—but make sure you're circling from your shoulders and not from your elbows.
4. Repeat Step 3 for 45 seconds.

Break: 15 seconds.

5. **SWAN**

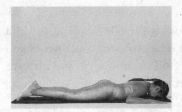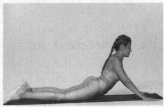

1. Lie prone on your stomach with your arms out by your side in a W. Your elbows should be in line with your shoulders and your legs should be straight. Make sure your pelvis is on the floor.
2. Inhale to engage the abdominals, slide your shoulder blades down your back and lift your chest off the mat into extension as you press your hands into the mat and look straight ahead. (Your elbows may or may not straighten depending on the amount of spinal extension that is safe and achievable for you.)
3. Lower your torso down with control.
4. Repeat Steps 2 and 3 for 45 seconds.

Break: 15 seconds.

*Repeat all five exercises to complete your 10-minute stack. Upper Body Stack 1 is done.*

## UPPER BODY STACK 2

Upper Body Stack 2 has five exercises. Each exercise will be done for 45 seconds with a 15-second break. Repeat once more to complete the 10-minute stack. You can either follow the steps below or use your phone to scan the QR code, and select

Upper Body Stack 2 from the menu to work out along with me. Wherever possible, an easier, modified version of the exercises is also available.

## 1. CRAWL TO MIDAS TOUCH

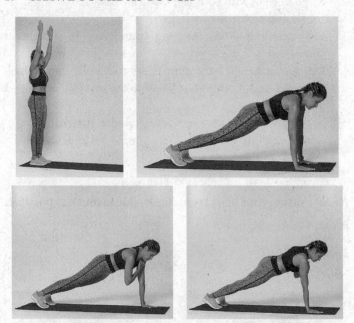

1. Stand upright with your feet hip-width apart.
2. Inhale and raise your arms up.
3. Exhale to roll down towards the floor, keeping your knees as straight as possible.

4. Using your hands, 'walk' into a plank in four counts, making sure your body is in a straight line from your head to your heels with shoulders directly above your wrists, abdominals engaged, glutes squeezed, your heels reaching away from you.
5. In this position, tap the opposite shoulder. Alternate.
6. 'Walk' back and roll yourself up.
7. Repeat Steps 1 to 6 for 45 seconds.

**Avoid shifting your body from side to side as much as possible.**

OR

## 1A. MODIFICATION: CRAWL TO MODIFIED PLANK

1. Stand upright with your feet hip-width apart.
2. Inhale and raise your arms up.
3. Exhale to roll down, keeping your knees as straight as you can.
4. Using your hands, bend your knees and 'walk' into a plank in four counts. Lower your knees to the mat to come into a modified plank.
5. In this position, tap the opposite shoulder. Alternate.
6. Come back into the plank, bend your knees and 'walk' back towards your feet and roll up.
7. Repeat Steps 1 to 6 for 45 seconds.

**Avoid shifting your body from side to side as much as possible.**

Break: 15 seconds.

## 2. CRAB LIFT

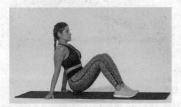 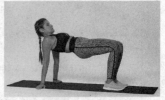

1. Sit on the mat with your knees bent and your arms behind you with your fingertips facing away from each other.
2. Draw your shoulders away from your ears.
3. Lift your hips off the mat towards the ceiling looking straight ahead and pulling your abdominals in.
4. Fold at the hips and lower down towards the mat for a split second and lift up again.
5. Repeat Step 4 for 45 seconds.

OR

## 2A. MODIFICATION: BRIDGE

1. Lie supine on the mat with your knees bent and feet flat on the mat.
2. Press into the feet and lift the hips towards the ceiling, keeping the shoulders on the mat.
3. Hold this position for 45 seconds.

Break: 15 seconds.

## 3. SIDE LYING TRICEPS

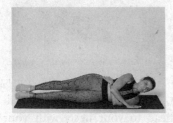 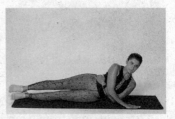

1. Lie on your side with your body in a straight line from your ear to your hip to your heel.
2. Your bottom hand is around your waist and the top hand is on the mat in front of you.

3. From here, press your top hand into the mat, and extend your elbow to lift your upper body up and bend again to lower down.
4. Repeat Step 3 for 45 seconds.

**Make sure you maintain your body in a straight line and don't allow your hips to move back and forth.**

OR
## 3A. MODIFICATION: MODIFIED SIDE LYING TRICEPS

1. For the modified version, repeat Steps 1 to 3 above, with the bottom knee bent and repeat the same movement for 45 seconds.

Break: 15 seconds.

## 4. CROUCH TO PLANK

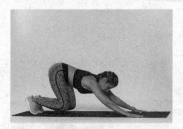 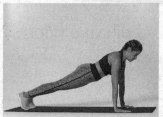

1. Start in the plank position. Make sure your body is in a straight line from your head to your heels with your shoulders directly above your wrists, abdominals engaged, glutes squeezed, your heels reaching away from you.
2. Press into your hands, and take your hips towards your heels, making sure that your hands are straight, and your head is between your arms.
3. Come back into a plank.
4. Repeat Steps 2 and 3 for 45 seconds.

OR

## 4A. MODIFICATION: CHILD POSE TO MODIFIED PLANK

1. Start in the child pose by sitting on the mat with your legs folded under you, hips touching your heels, arms reaching in front of you on the mat, and shoulders away from the ears.
2. Without moving your hands, come forward into a modified plank with your wrists under your shoulders and knees on the mat. Make sure your body is in a straight line from your head to your knees.
3. Repeat Steps 1 and 2 for 45 seconds.

Break: 15 seconds

## 5. SWIMMING

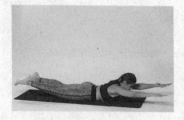 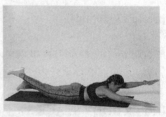

1. Lie prone on your stomach. Your arms and legs should be reaching away from each other. Think of your toes and fingertips being in opposition, pulling away from each other.
2. Engage your abdominals, squeeze your glutes and pull your shoulders away from your ears.
3. Reach one leg and the opposite arm out and up towards the ceiling. Switch the arm and leg quickly without losing the balance on the centre of the torso. Breathe in the pattern of two inhalations followed by two exhalations.
4. Repeat Step 3 for 45 seconds.

**Try to keep your torso completely stable by continuing to engage your abdominals and squeezing your glutes.**

OR

## 5A. MODIFICATION: ALTERNATE ARM AND LEG LIFT

1. Lie prone on your stomach. Your arms and legs should be reaching away from each other. Think of your toes and fingertips being in opposition, pulling away from each other.
2. Engage your abdominals, squeeze your glutes and pull your shoulders away from your ears.
3. Lift the opposite arm and leg and lower them. Alternate with the other side.
4. Repeat Step 3 for 45 seconds.

Break: 15 seconds.

*Repeat all five exercises to complete your 10-minute stack. Upper Body Stack 2 is done.*

## UPPER BODY STACK 3

Upper Body Stack 3 has five exercises. Each exercise will be done for 45 seconds with a 15-second break. Repeat once more to complete the 10-minute stack. You can either follow the steps below or use your phone to scan the QR code, and select Upper Body Stack 3 from the menu to  work out along with me. Wherever possible, an easier, modified version of the exercises is also available.

## 1. PLANK TO T

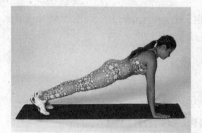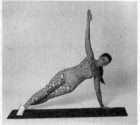

1. Start in the plank position. Make sure your body is in a straight line from your head to your heels with your shoulders directly above your wrists, abdominals engaged, glutes squeezed, and your heels reaching away from you.
2. From this position, rotate your legs and body to the side and stretch your free hand to the ceiling to form a T.
3. Come back into the plank position.
4. Rotate to the other side.
5. Repeat Steps 3 and 4 for 45 seconds, and keep alternating sides.

**Do this exercise in a flow.**

OR

## 1A. MODIFICATION: MODIFIED PLANK TO T

1. Lie prone on the floor. Position your arms under your shoulders and press into your arms to come up into a modified plank. Keep your knees on the floor and your body in a straight line from your head to your knees with your shoulders directly above your wrists, your abdominals engaged and glutes squeezed.
2. From this position, rotate to the side, straighten the top leg, keeping your other knee stable on the mat and stretch your free hand to the ceiling to form a T.

3. Come back into the modified plank position. Rotate to the other side.
4. Repeat Steps 2 and 3 for 45 seconds, and keep alternating sides.

**Do this exercise in a flow.**

Break: 15 seconds.

2. **SEATED TRICEPS DIPS TO HIP LIFT**

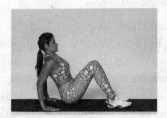 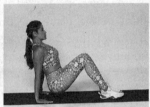

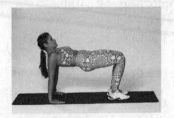

1. Sit on the mat with your knees bent, hands behind you and fingers pointing towards your feet.
2. Lift your hips off the mat into crab position with your elbows straight and shoulders away from your ears.
3. From this position, bend your elbows to lower your hips towards the floor and as you extend them, lift your hips up back into crab position.
4. Repeat Step 3 for 45 seconds.

OR
## 2A. MODIFICATION: SEATED TRICEPS DIPS

For the modified version, do the Seated Triceps Dips without going into the crab position. You will find the steps on page 90.

Repeat for 45 seconds.

Break: 15 seconds.

## 3.   STANDING THUMBS DOWN PULSE

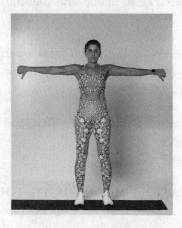

1.  Stand upright with your feet hip-width apart.
2.  Extend your arms out by your side in a T.
3.  Rotate your thumbs down, and pulse.
4.  The breath pattern is inhale-inhale, exhale-exhale, as you pulse.
5.  Repeat Steps 3 and 4 for 45 seconds.

Break: 15 seconds.

## 4.  ALL-FOURS TRICEPS PRESS

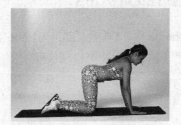 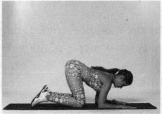

1.  Start in the all-fours position with your wrists in line with your shoulders, knees in line with your hips and your back neutral.
2.  Draw your shoulders down your back.
3.  Bend your elbows to lower your torso towards the floor and extend to come back to the starting position.
4.  Repeat Step 3 for 45 seconds.

**Remember to keep pressing into the floor, and keep your hips and knees stable.**

OR

## 4A. MODIFICATION: MODIFIED ALL-FOURS TRICEPS PRESS

To modify, make the triceps press a bit shallow and repeat for 45 seconds.

Break: 15 seconds.

## 5.   SEATED SPINE TWIST

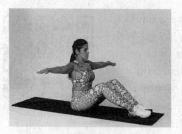 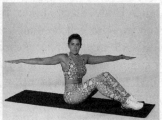

1. Sit on the floor with your legs in a diamond position—knees bent, feet pressed together. Keep your spine upright, sitting on the centre of your sit bones.
2. Extend your arms out by your side in a T with your palms facing down.
3. From this position, root both sit bones into the ground and rotate the torso to the right keeping the arms directly out to the side. Pulse twice in the rotation and return to the centre. Rotate to the other side.
4. Repeat Step 3 for 45 seconds.

**Remember to keep elongating your spine.**

OR

## 5A. MODIFICATION: SEATED SPINE TWIST WITH ARMS BENT

To modify, interlace your fingers and place them behind your head at the nape of your neck. Press your head into your hands, and follow Step 3 above for 45 seconds.

Break: 15 seconds.

*Repeat all five exercises to complete your 10-minute stack. Upper Body Stack 3 is done.*

## UPPER BODY STACK 4

Upper Body Stack 4 has five exercises. Each exercise will be done for 45 seconds with a 15-second break. Repeat once more to complete the 10-minute stack. You can either follow the steps below or use your phone to scan the QR code, and select Upper Body Stack 4 from the menu to  work out along with me. Wherever possible, an easier, modified version of the exercises is also available.

### 1.  CRAWL TO PUSH-UP

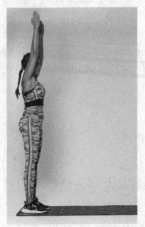 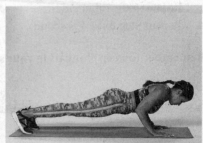

1.  Stand upright with your feet hip-width apart.
2.  Inhale and raise your arms up.
3.  Exhale to roll down towards the floor, keeping your knees as straight as possible.
4.  Using your hands, 'walk' into a plank in four counts. Make sure your body is in a straight line from your head to your heels with your shoulders directly above your wrists,

abdominals engaged, glutes squeezed, and your heels reaching away from you.

5. Do a push-up by bending your elbows and lowering your body towards the mat. Extend your elbows and use your triceps to push back up into the plank position.

6. Go into a pike by pushing your hips up towards the ceiling and 'walk' your hands back towards your feet to roll up to the starting position mentioned in (1).

7. Repeat Steps 1 to 6 for 45 seconds.

OR

## 1A. MODIFICATION: CRAWL TO KNEE PUSH-UP

1. Stand upright with your feet hip-width apart.

2. Inhale and raise your arms up.

3. Exhale to roll down, keeping your knees as straight as you can.

4. Using your hands, bend your knees and 'walk' into the plank position in four counts. Lower your knees to the mat to come into a modified plank.

5. Make sure your body is in a straight line from your head to your knees.

6. Do a knee push-up by bending your elbows and lowering your body towards the mat. Extend your elbows and use your triceps to push back up into a modified plank.

7. Lifting your knees off the mat, come back into the plank position, bend your knees and 'walk' back towards your feet and roll up.

8. Repeat Steps 1 to 7 for 45 seconds.

Break: 15 seconds.

## 2.　CRAB MARCHING

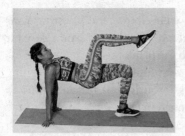 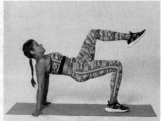

1.  Sit on the mat with your knees bent and your arms behind you with your fingertips facing away from each other.
2.  Draw your shoulders away from your ears.
3.  Lift your hips off the mat towards the ceiling. Look straight ahead, pull your abdominals in and squeeze your glutes.
4.  From this position, pressing into one foot, lift the other leg and lower it down. Change legs.
5.  Repeat Step 4 for 45 seconds.

**Try to keep your upper body and hips stable as you move your legs.**

OR
## 2A. MODIFICATION: CRAB

For the modified version, follow Steps 1 to 3 above to go into the crab position, and come back down. Tap your hips to the floor and come back up again. Repeat for 45 seconds.

Break: 15 seconds.

### 3.  PRONE THUMBS-UP PULSES

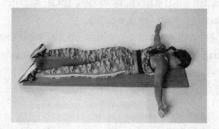

1. Lie prone on your stomach with your arms out by your side in a T.
2. Your elbows should be in line with your shoulders, your legs should be straight, and your pelvis should be on the floor.
3. Rotate your thumbs towards the ceiling and pulse your thumbs up for 45 seconds.
4. Breathe in the pattern of inhale-inhale, exhale-exhale, as you pulse.

**Make sure you draw your shoulders down.**

Break: 15 seconds.

### 4.  ALL-FOURS HOVER TO PIKE

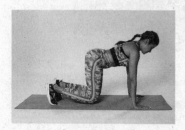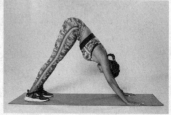

1. Start in the all-fours position with your wrists in line with your shoulders and knees in line with your hips. Draw your

shoulders down your back and, pressing into your hands and toes, lift your knees, hovering them slightly off the mat, while keeping your back neutral.

2. From this position, tilt your hips up, lifting them up towards the ceiling into the pike position, while lowering your heels.
3. Return to the all-fours hover.
4. Repeat Steps 2 and 3 for 45 seconds.

OR

## 4A. MODIFICATION: ALL-FOURS TO PIKE

1. The knees won't hover in the modified version.
2. From the all-fours position mentioned in Step 1 above, lift your hips to the ceiling into the pike position, lowering your heels. Come back on all-fours, resting your knees on the mat.
3. Repeat Step 2 for 45 seconds.

Break: 15 seconds.

## 5.  ROCKET

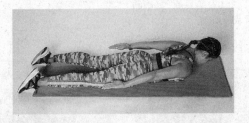

1. Lie prone face down with your arms by your side and palms facing the ceiling.
2. Engage your abdominals and squeeze your glutes.
3. Take a breath and lift your head, shoulders and chest off the mat.
4. Pulse your palms up, breathing in a pattern of inhale-inhale, exhale-exhale, for 45 seconds.

**Keep engaging your abdominals and squeezing your glutes. Keep your knees straight and look at the front edge of your mat.**

Break: 15 seconds.

*Repeat all five exercises to complete your 10-minute stack. Upper Body Stack 4 is done.*

## UPPER BODY STACK 5

Upper Body Stack 5 has five exercises. Each exercise will be done for 45 seconds with a 15-second break. Repeat once more to complete the 10-minute stack. You can either follow the steps below or use your phone to scan the QR code, and select Upper Body Stack 5 from the menu to work out along with me. Wherever possible, an easier, modified version of the exercises is also available.

1. **SQUAT WITH UPPER CUT, UPPER CUT, PUNCH, PUNCH**

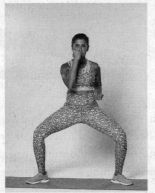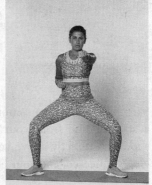

1. Start in a wide squat with your legs wide, toes turned out and knees directly over your toes.
2. Pull your abdominals in, and make sure that you're upright in this position.
3. Punch up (upper cut) with each hand, and then punch forward (punch). Follow the pattern of upper cut, upper cut, punch, punch.
4. Maintaining the squat, repeat Step 3 for 45 seconds.

**Make sure that your body doesn't sway from side to side.**

OR

**1A. MODIFICATION: STANDING UPPER CUT, UPPER CUT, PUNCH, PUNCH**

For the modified version, do the same as above in a standing position; don't squat. Repeat for 45 seconds.

Break: 15 seconds.

**2. SUICIDE PUSH**

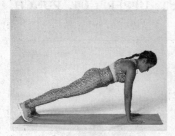 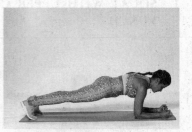

1. Start in the plank position. Make sure your body is in a straight line from your head to your heels with your shoulders directly above your wrists, abdominals engaged, glutes squeezed, and your heels reaching away from you.

2.  From this position, bend your elbows and lower your body on to your forearms to get into a forearm plank.
3.  Extend your elbows and push yourself back up into the plank position, one hand at a time, using the palm to press into the floor.
4.  Keep alternating between plank and forearm plank for 45 seconds.

**Keep your torso and hips stable when alternating between plank and forearm plank.**

OR
## 2A. MODIFICATION: SUICIDE PUSH ON KNEES

For the modified version, do the same exercise but in the all-fours position (you can follow the form on page 102). Keep your hips stable, and do this for 45 seconds.

Break: 15 seconds.

## 3.   RHOMBOIDS WITH ALTERNATE KNEE LIFT

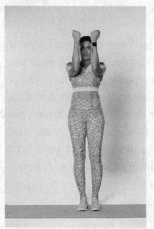 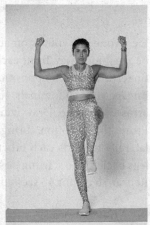

1. Stand upright with your feet closer than hip-width apart.
2. Bend your elbows and keep your hands in front of you with your palms facing you. Your elbows should be in line with your shoulders.
3. From this position, open both your elbows out to the side, simultaneously lifting one knee.
4. Bring your elbows back to the centre, simultaneously placing your foot back down.
5. Lift your other knee, and open your elbows again, and keep repeating the movement as you alternate with the knees for 45 seconds.

Break: 15 seconds.

4. **REVERSE ANGELS**

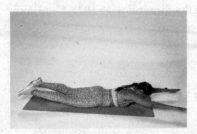 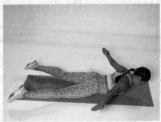

1. Lie prone on your stomach. Your arms and legs should be reaching away from each other. Think of your toes and fingertips being in opposition, pulling away from each other.
2. Engage your abdominals, squeeze your glutes and float your arms and legs up. Draw your shoulders away from your ears.
3. From this position, bring (abduct) your arms and legs laterally towards each other and then move your arms and legs back to the starting position (adduct) and repeat.
4. Repeat Step 3 for 45 seconds.

Break: 15 seconds.

## 5. PLANK KNEE DRIVE TO PIKE

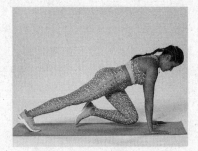 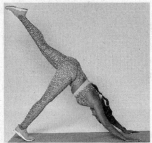

1. Start in the plank position. Make sure your body is in a straight line from your head to your heels with your shoulders directly above your wrists, abdominals engaged, glutes squeezed, and your heels reaching away from you.
2. Bring one knee to your chest and then take that foot straight up towards the ceiling. Bring the same knee to the chest again.
3. Repeat Step 2 for 20 seconds and switch sides for a total of 45 seconds.

OR

### 5A. MODIFICATION: PLANK TO PIKE

For the modified version, come into the plank position as in Step 1 above and go into a pike, i.e., push your hips towards the ceiling as far you can. Come back into the plank position again and repeat this movement for 45 seconds.

Break: 15 seconds.

*Repeat all five exercises to complete your 10-minute stack.*
*Upper Body Stack 5 is done.*

# 10-Minute Lower Body Stacks

10-Minute Lower Body Stacks

## LOWER BODY STACK 1

Lower Body Stack 1 has five exercises. Each exercise will be done for 45 seconds with a 15-second break. Repeat once more to complete the 10-minute stack. You can either follow the steps below or use your phone to scan the QR code, and select  Lower Body Stack 1 from the menu to work out along with me.

### 1. SQUAT

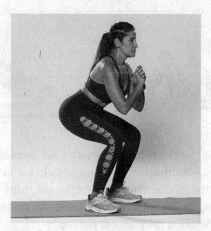

1. Stand upright with your feet slightly wider than shoulder-width apart and toes slightly turned out.
2. Engage your abdominals, flex at the hips, and push them back and lower down as if sitting on an invisible chair. Let your knees follow the direction of your feet, without extending over your toes.

3.  Straighten up to the standing position by extending your legs. Squeeze your glutes at the top, without thrusting the hips forward.
4.  Repeat Steps 2 and 3 for 45 seconds.

**Keep your back neutral and chest open throughout the movement.**

**This is a basic squat. To make this more challenging, you can add dumbbells or waterbells. But do make sure that your knees don't extend over your toes.**

Break: 15 seconds.

### 2. BRIDGE

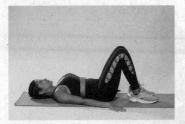 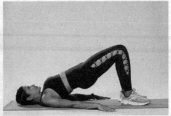

1.  Lie supine (face up) on the mat with your knees bent, your feet flat and hip-width apart, and your arms in a V at your sides.
2.  Engage the abdominals and press the hips up towards the ceiling to lift your back off the floor keeping the spine neutral. Squeeze the glutes at the top.
3.  Lower the hips back to the mat with control.
4.  Repeat Steps 2 and 3 for 45 seconds.

Break: 15 seconds.

### 3.  ALTERNATE REVERSE LUNGE

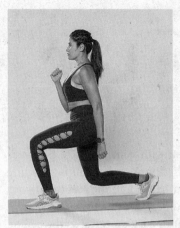 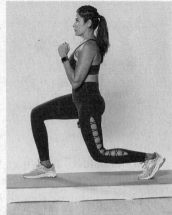

1.  Stand upright with your feet hip-width apart.
2.  Step back with your right foot, lowering it down towards the floor as you bend the left knee. Your left thigh should be almost parallel to the floor.
3.  Pressing your left heel into the floor, return to the standing position by bringing your right leg forward.
4.  Alternate legs, stepping back with the left leg.
5.  Keep alternating legs for 45 seconds.

**To make it easier, keep your hands on your waist if you don't want to move them. To make it more challenging, you can add dumbbells or waterbells.**

Break: 15 seconds.

## 4.  ALL-FOURS BUTT BLASTER

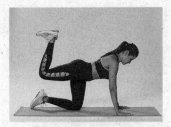

1.  Start in the all-fours position with your wrists in line with your shoulders and knees in line with your hips. Keeping your back neutral, press your hands into the mat to lift your chest up and draw your shoulders down your back.
2.  Keeping your hips stable, lift one leg up towards the ceiling with your foot flexed, and bring it back down to hover over the mat and take it back up.
3.  Repeat for 20 seconds and switch sides for a total of 45 seconds.

**Keep your torso stable as you move your leg.**

Break: 15 seconds.

## 5.  RUNNING IN PLACE

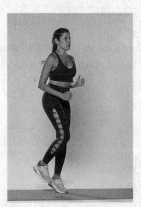
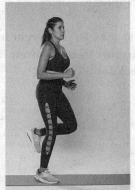

1. Stand upright with your feet slightly closer than hip-width apart.
2. Lift alternate knees up to run in place for 45 seconds.

Break: 15 seconds.

*Repeat all five exercises to complete your 10-minute stack.*
*Lower Body Stack 1 is done.*

## LOWER BODY STACK 2

Lower Body Stack 2 has five exercises. Each exercise will be done for 45 seconds with a 15-second break. Repeat once more to complete the 10-minute stack. You can either follow the steps below or use your phone to scan the QR code, and select  Lower Body Stack 2 from the menu to work out along with me. Wherever possible, an easier, modified version of the exercises is also available.

### 1. DOUBLE PULSE SUMO SQUAT

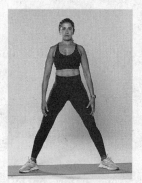 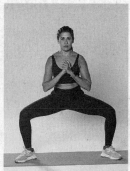

1. Stand upright with your feet much wider than shoulder-width apart and toes turned out.

2. Engage your abdominals, flex at the hips, push them back and lower down as if sitting on an invisible chair. Let your knees follow the direction of your feet, without extending over your toes.

3. Pulse down for two counts and straighten up by extending your legs. Squeeze your glutes at the top, without thrusting the hips forward.

4. Repeat Steps 2 and 3 for 45 seconds.

**Keep your back neutral and your chest open throughout the movement.**

**To make this more challenging, you can add dumbbells or waterbells.**

OR
## 1A. MODIFICATION: SUMO SQUAT

For the modified version, squat as above but don't pulse. Just go up and down for 45 seconds.

Break: 15 seconds.

## 2. DECLINE KNEE DRIVE

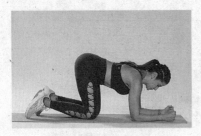 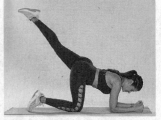

1. Come into the all-fours position on your forearms by bending the elbows and placing them directly under your shoulders with your forearms on the mat in line with the elbows.

2. Pressing your forearms into the mat, lift your chest up and slide your shoulders down your back, engaging the abdominals.
3. Bring one knee towards your chest and drive the same leg straight up towards the ceiling, keeping your shoulders stable by pressing equally into both forearms. Bring your knee to your chest again.
4. Repeat Step 3 for 20 seconds and switch sides for a total of 45 seconds.

OR

**2A. MODIFICATION: ALL-FOURS KNEE DRIVE**

For the modified version, come into the all-fours position and follow Steps 3 and 4 above for 45 seconds. Do not come on to your forearms.

Break: 15 seconds.

**3.   ALTERNATE FORWARD LUNGE**

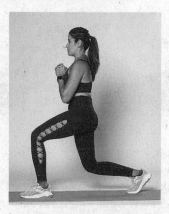

1. Stand upright with your feet hip-width apart.
2. Take a step forward with your left foot and bend the right knee. Your left thigh should be almost parallel to the floor.

3.  Pressing into your left foot, return to the standing position by bringing your left leg back.
4.  Alternate legs, stepping forward with the right leg, and come back.
5.  Keep alternating legs for 45 seconds.

**To make this more challenging, you can add dumbbells or water bells.**

OR
## 3A. MODIFICATION: STATIONARY LUNGE

For a modified version, go into a stationary lunge. Take one step forward and bend the knee of the other leg to come into a front lunge. Bend and straighten the back leg for 20 seconds and switch legs for a total of 45 seconds.

Break: 15 seconds.

## 4.  CLAM

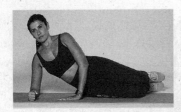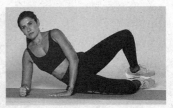

1.  Lie on your side on your forearm with your elbow in line with your shoulders.
2.  Press your forearm into the mat to engage your lats, sliding your shoulder away from your ears.
3.  Keeping your knees in line with your hips, fold them at a ninety-degree angle, placing your feet behind you.
4.  The other hand can be either on the mat or around your waist.

5. Making sure your hips are stacked on top of each other and, keeping your feet together, lift and lower the top knee without disturbing the alignment of the hips and shoulders. You should feel this exercise in your glutes.

6. Repeat Step 5 for 20 seconds and switch sides for a total of 45 seconds.

OR

## 4A. MODIFICATION: MODIFIED CLAM

To modify this exercise, change the starting position by bringing your knees forward and keeping your heels in line with your glutes. Do the rest of the exercise as usual for 45 seconds, changing sides halfway through.

Break: 15 seconds.

## 5. SPIDERMAN CLIMB

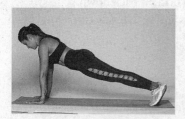
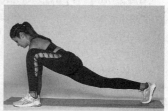
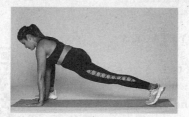

1. Start in the plank position with your wrists under your shoulders. Press into your hands to lift your chest and open it. Engage your abdominals, squeeze your glutes, and reach your heels away from you.
2. From this position, bring one leg next to your hand on the same side, dropping your hips down. Come back to the plank position, and switch with the other leg. Keep alternating legs for 45 seconds.

OR

**5A. MODIFICATION: FIRE HYDRANT**

1. Get into the all-fours position with your wrists in line with your shoulders and knees in line with your hips. Keeping your back neutral, press into your hands to lift your shoulders away from the mat.
2. Keeping the ninety-degree angle of your leg, engage your abdominals and lift your knee sideways as perpendicular to the ground as possible, and bring it back down.
3. Repeat Step 2 for 20 seconds and switch sides for a total of 45 seconds.

Break: 15 seconds.

*Repeat all five exercises to complete your 10-minute stack.*
*Lower Body Stack 2 is done.*

**LOWER BODY STACK 3**

Lower Body Stack 3 has five exercises. Each exercise will be done for 45 seconds with a 15-second break. Repeat once more to complete the 10-minute stack. You can either follow the steps below or use your

phone to scan the QR code, and select Lower Body Stack 3 from the menu to work out along with me. Wherever possible, an easier, modified version of the exercises is also available.

## 1.  SINGLE LEG SQUAT

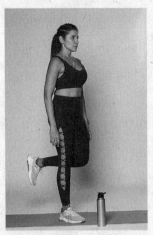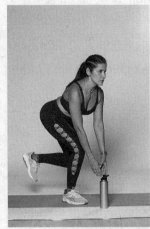

1.  Place a bottle in front of you.
2.  Stand directly behind it.
3.  Engage your core and, lifting one foot off the mat, flex at the hips and lower them down to the imaginary chair behind you, and touch the bottle. Come back to the standing position by extending your knee.
4.  Repeat Step 3 for 20 seconds and switch sides for a total of 45 seconds.

**Don't forget to keep your back neutral. As this is a squat, remember to use your gluteal muscles.**

OR
## 1A. MODIFICATION: SQUAT

To modify, hold the bottle in your hands and simply squat. You can follow the instructions for a squat on page 117. Hold this position for 45 seconds.

Break: 15 seconds.

## 2. ALTERNATE REVERSE LUNGE

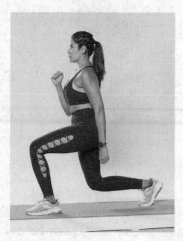
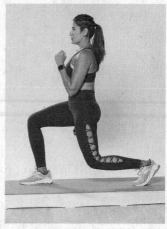

1. Stand upright with your feet hip-width apart.
2. Step back with your right foot, lowering it down towards the floor as you bend the left knee.
3. Your left thigh should be almost parallel to the floor.
4. Pressing your left heel into the floor, return to the standing position by bringing your right leg forward.
5. Alternate legs, stepping back with the left foot.
6. Keep alternating legs for 45 seconds.

**Don't forget to lengthen your body and try not to slouch.**

Break: 15 seconds.

## 3.  ALL-FOURS FIRE HYDRANT

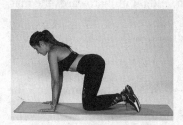 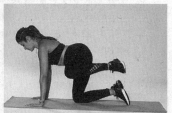

1.  Form the all-fours position with your wrists in line with your shoulders and knees in line with your hips. Keeping your back neutral, press into your hands to lift your shoulders away from the mat.
2.  Keeping the ninety-degree angle of your leg, engage your abdominals and lift your knee sideways as perpendicular to the ground as possible, and bring it back down.
3.  Repeat Step 2 for 20 seconds and switch sides for a total of 45 seconds.

Break: 15 seconds.

## 4.  LOW PULSE LUNGES

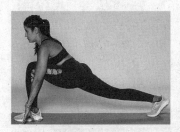 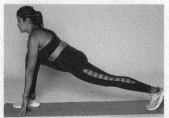

1. Stand upright on the mat. Take a big step back with one leg to go into a deep lunge. Place both your hands on either side of the front foot, keeping the back leg straight. Try to keep your chest up.
2. Maintaining this position, pulse down and up, making sure to keep your hip flexor open, and pointing towards the mat. Keep pulsing.
3. Repeat Step 2 for 20 seconds and switch sides for a total of 45 seconds.

**Don't allow the front knee to go over the toes, and keep the back leg as straight as possible.**

OR

**4A. MODIFICATION: DEEP LUNGE HOLD**

For the modified version, hold the deep lunge for 20 seconds. This is an isometric exercise that will enable your hip flexor to gain some strength. Switch legs after 20 seconds for a total of 45 seconds.

Break: 15 seconds.

**5.   LATERAL SQUAT WALK**

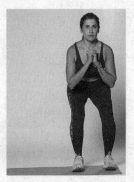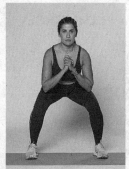

1. Stand upright with your feet shoulder-width apart.
2. Flex at the hips with a neutral back and engage your abdominals as you lower down into a squat.
3. From this position, take a step to the side. Take as many steps to the same side as the space you have. Take equal steps on the other side. Repeat for 45 seconds.

OR

## 5A. MODIFICATION: SQUAT

For a modified version, do a simple squat (page 117) so that you can gain strength and build up to the lateral squat walk.

Break: 15 seconds.

*Repeat all five exercises to complete your 10-minute stack.*
*Lower Body Stack 3 is done.*

## LOWER BODY STACK 4

Lower Body Stack 4 has five exercises. Each exercise will be done for 45 seconds with a 15-second break. Repeat once more to complete the 10-minute stack. You can either follow the steps below or use your phone to scan the QR code, and select  Lower Body Stack 4 from the menu to work out along with me. Wherever possible, an easier, modified version of the exercises is also available.

### 1. MOVING SQUATS

1. Stand upright with your feet together and pull up your pelvic floor.

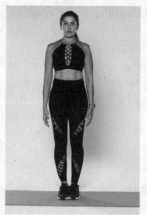 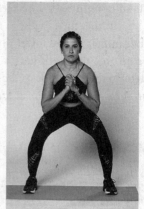

2.  From this position, take a step to the side and engage your abdominals, flex at the hips to squat and come back to the centre upright.
3.  In the same way, squat to the other side and come back to the centre upright.
4.  Keep alternating sides for 45 seconds.

OR

**1A. MODIFICATION: SQUAT**

To modify this exercise, do a regular squat (steps on page 117), and come back up. Squat and stand up for 45 seconds.

**If your knee hurts, you can do a slightly wider squat by increasing the distance between your feet. This takes the pressure off your knees.**

Break: 15 seconds.

## 2.  LATERAL LUNGES

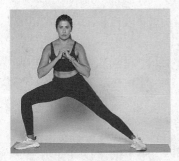 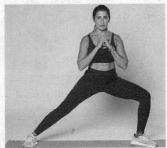

1.  Stand upright with your feet hip-width apart.
2.  Engage your core and step out laterally. Now, shift your weight and bend the knee to go into a side lunge. Keep the knee in the direction of the toes and don't allow it to extend over the toes.
3.  Engaging your core, press into that foot to lift it, and return to the starting position.
4.  Repeat Steps 2 and 3 for 20 seconds and switch sides for a total of 45 seconds.

OR
## 2A. MODIFICATION: LATERAL SIDE STEPS

1.  Stand upright with your feet hip-width apart, step out to the side and come back.
2.  Repeat Step 1 for 20 seconds and switch sides for a total of 45 seconds.

Break: 15 seconds

## 3.  PRONE FROG LIFTS

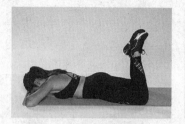 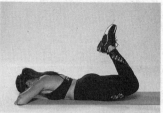

1.  Lie prone (face down) on the mat with your hands under your forehead. Draw your shoulders down your back, engage your abdominals, and tuck your pelvis under you to make sure that you're not overextending your lower back.
2.  Bend your knees and bring your feet together to form a diamond (also known as the frog position).
3.  Lift and lower your thighs and knees off the mat, squeezing your glutes and keeping your heels together.
4.  Repeat Step 3 for 45 seconds.

OR

## 3A. MODIFICATION: PRONE ALTERNATE STRAIGHT LEG LIFTS

1.  Lie prone on the mat with your hands under your hips and elbows on the mat.
2.  Drawing your shoulders down your back,  alternately lift the (straight) legs for 45 seconds.

Break: 15 seconds.

## 4.  FORWARD AND REVERSE LUNGE

1.  Stand upright with your feet hip-width apart.

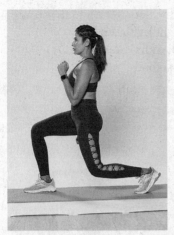 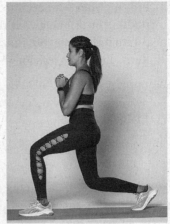

2.  Step forward with your right foot, lowering it down towards the floor as you bend the left knee. Your right thigh should be almost parallel to the floor.

3.  Pressing into your right foot, return to the standing position by bringing your right leg back and immediately step back with your right foot, lowering it down towards the floor as you bend the left knee. Your left thigh should be almost parallel to the floor.

4.  Pressing your left heel into the floor, return to the standing position by bringing your right leg forward.

5.  Repeat Steps 2 to 4 for 20 seconds and switch sides for a total of 45 seconds.

OR
## 4A. MODIFICATION: ALTERNATE REVERSE LUNGE

1.  Stand upright with your feet hip-width apart.

2.  Step back with your right foot, lowering it down towards the floor as you bend the left knee. Your left thigh should be almost parallel to the floor.

3. Pressing your left heel into the floor, return to the standing position by bringing your right leg forward.
4. Alternate legs, stepping back with the left foot.
5. Keep alternating legs for 45 seconds.

Break: 15 seconds.

## 5.  CIRCLE KICKS

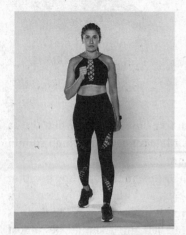
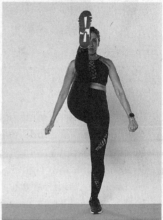
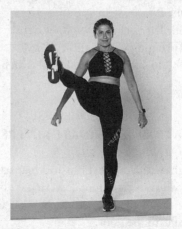

1. Stand upright with your feet hip-width apart.
2. Take one leg back across your body in a circle and return to the starting position. Try to keep your legs as straight as possible.
3. Repeat Step 2 for 20 seconds and switch sides for a total of 45 seconds.

OR
## 5A. MODIFICATION: STANDING HIP CIRCLES

1. Stand upright with your feet hip-width apart.
2. Take one leg back, lift the foot off the floor, bending at the knee and circling clockwise at the hip to return to the starting position. Make the circle as big as possible.
3. Repeat Step 2 for 20 seconds and switch sides for a total of 45 seconds.

Break: 15 seconds.

*Repeat all five exercises to complete your 10-minute stack.*
*Lower Body Stack 4 is done.*

## LOWER BODY STACK 5

Lower Body Stack 5 has five exercises. Each exercise will be done for 45 seconds with a 15-second break. Repeat once more to complete the 10-minute stack. You can either follow the steps below or use your phone to scan the QR code, and select  Lower Body Stack 5 from the menu to work out along with me. Wherever possible, an easier, modified version of the exercises is also available.

## 1. SQUAT AND SIDE LEG LIFT

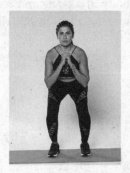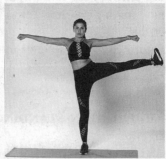

1. Stand upright with your feet hip-width apart and toes slightly turned out.
2. Engage your abdominals, flex at the hips, push them back, and lower down as if sitting on an invisible chair. Let your knees follow the direction of your feet, without extending over your toes.
3. Extend your legs to straighten up, lift one leg out laterally to the side and lower it on to the mat.
4. Squat once more, and lift the other leg out laterally.
5. Repeat Steps 2 to 4 for 45 seconds.

**Keep your back neutral throughout the movement and your chest open.**

OR
**1A. MODIFICATION: SQUAT**

1. Do a simple squat (steps on page 117).
2. Repeat for 45 seconds.

Break: 15 seconds.

## 2.   SIDE KNEELING KICKS

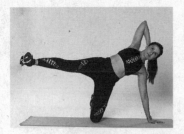 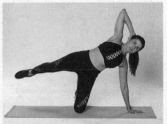

1.   Kneel on the mat, with your arms stretched out to your sides in a T.
2.   Lean over to one side until the hand touches the mat, with the opposite knee off the mat and the leg at hip level.
3.   Press into the mat to activate your lats and draw your shoulders away from your ears. Place the top hand behind your head.
4.   Flex your foot and kick forward for two counts, point your foot and take the leg back. Flex and kick, point and back.
5.   Repeat Step 4 for 20 seconds and switch sides for a total of 45 seconds.

OR
## 2A. MODIFICATION: SIDE LYING KICKS

1.   Lie on your side with your body in a straight line from your ear to your hip and take your legs slightly forward. Lift your torso, prop your head up with your bottom hand, and place your top hand on the floor in front of you.
2.   Flex the top foot and kick forward for two counts, point your foot and take the leg back. Flex and kick, point and back.
3.   Repeat Step 2 for 20 seconds and switch sides for a total of 45 seconds.

Break: 15 seconds.

## 3.  CURTSY LUNGE

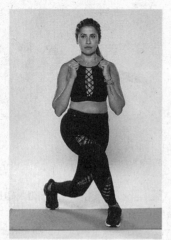 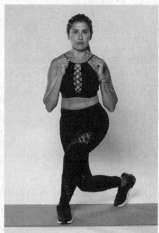

1.  Stand upright with your feet hip-width apart.
2.  Engage your core, take one leg diagonally across the back of the other and bend the knee to go into a lunge.
3.  Come back to the starting position, and repeat with the other leg.
4.  Make sure your body is upright. Don't lean forward and go as deep as you can without feeling discomfort in your knees.
5.  Alternate legs for 45 seconds.

OR
### 3A. MODIFICATION: ALTERNATE REVERSE LUNGE

To modify, you can do alternate reverse lunges (steps on page 119). This will help you build enough strength to attempt the curtsy lunges.

Break: 15 seconds.

## 4.  SINGLE LEG BRIDGE

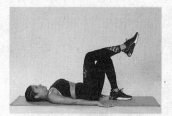 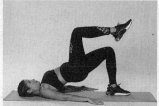

1.  Lie supine (face up) with your knees bent, feet flat on the mat and hip-width apart, with your arms in a V at the sides of your body.
2.  Lift one leg to the table-top position (also called 90/90), making sure that the knee is directly over your hip and that your calf is parallel to the floor.
3.  Press into your triceps to open your chest out and look straight at the ceiling.
4.  Engage your core and lift your hips towards the ceiling, and lower down keeping your hips square.
5.  Repeat Step 4 for 20 seconds and switch sides for a total of 45 seconds.


OR
## 4A. MODIFICATION: BRIDGE

To modify, you can go into a simple bridge (steps on page 118), and lift your hips up and lower them down for 45 seconds. Take care to press your triceps into the mat so that your upper body is stable as your lower body moves.

Break: 15 seconds.

## 5.    SQUAT AND JUMP

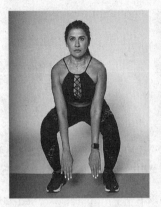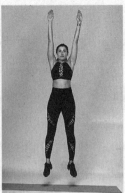

1.    Stand upright with your feet hip-width apart.
2.    Flex at the hips, lower into a squat and try to touch the floor, making sure you don't round your back.
3.    From this position, propel your body up and jump, raising your hands towards the ceiling.
4.    Repeat Steps 2 and 3 for 45 seconds.

OR
## 5A. MODIFICATION: SQUAT AND HEEL LIFT

This exercise can be made easier by squatting (steps on page 117) and lifting up your heels when you come back up with your back upright, and your hands raised towards the ceiling. Repeat for 45 seconds.

Break: 15 seconds.

*Repeat all five exercises to complete your 10-minute stack. Lower Body Stack 5 is done.*

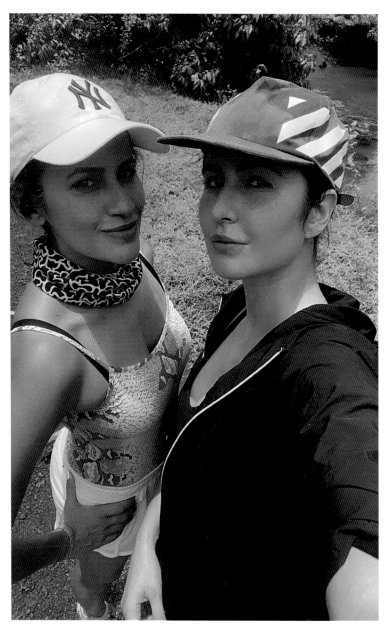

Katrina's peaceful workout look.
The calm before the storm!

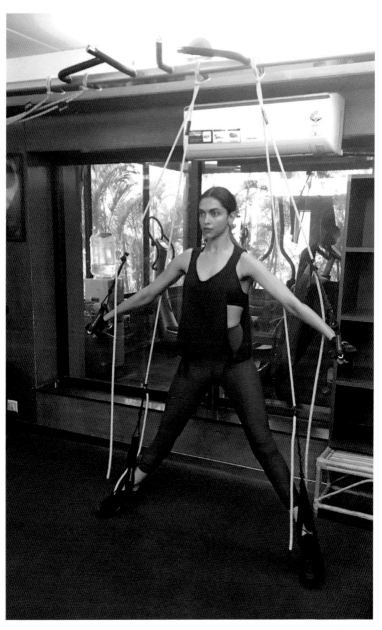

True to form, Deepika executing a perfect Four-Point Jack on the Bodhi
Pilates apparatus.

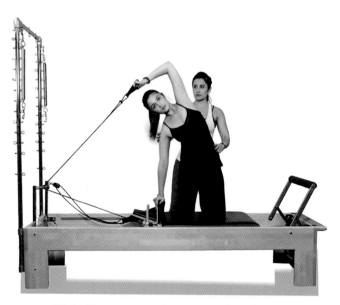

Alia looking to try something new on the Reformer.

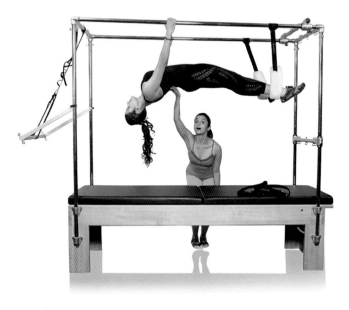

Alia supervising my Hanging Back Extension on the Trapeze.
The student becomes the master.

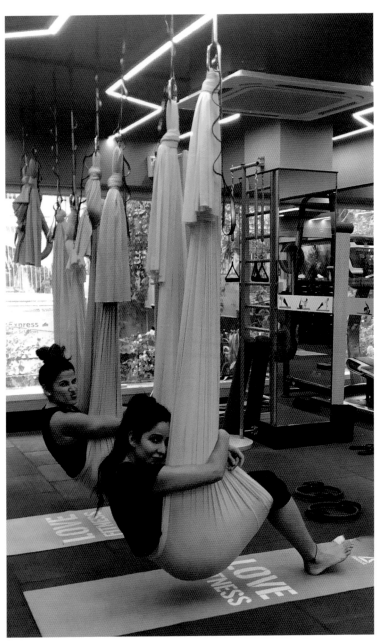

Hanging with Katrina and her injured toe.

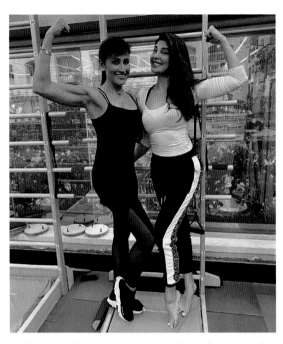

My biceps are bigger than yours, says Jacqueline Fernandes.

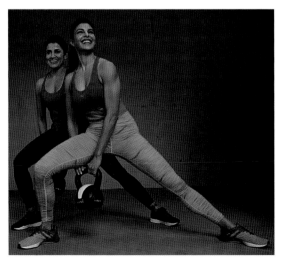

Jacqueline Fernandes smiling through some gruelling
Kettlebell Side Lunges.

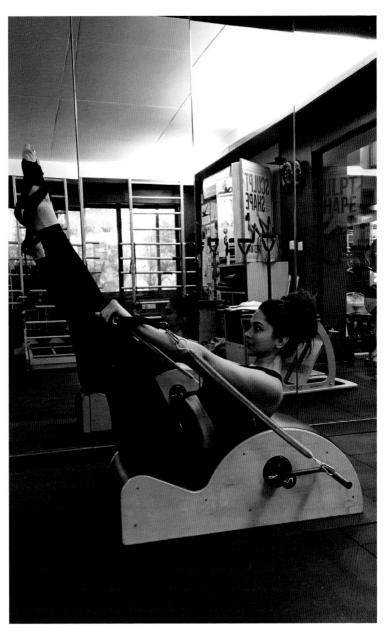

Focus, concentration and perfection are some words to describe Deepika's Teaser on the Spine Corrector.

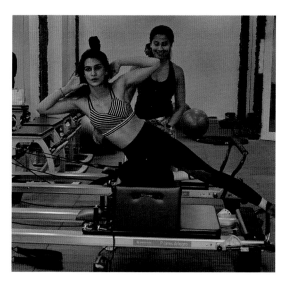

Mermaid on the Reformer, Kriti Sanon.

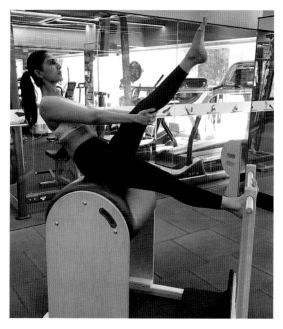

Vaani Kapoor climbs a tree on the Ladder Barrel when she can't do it outdoors.

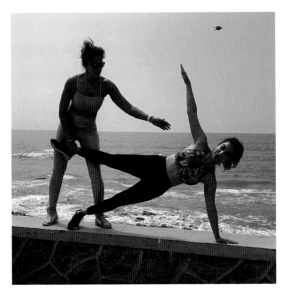

Why do something ordinary when you can make Sophie do a Single Leg Side Plank at Bandra Bandstand?

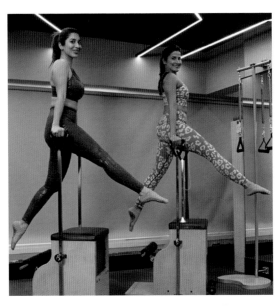

Sophie ready to take off on the Combo Chair.

# 10-Minute Abdominal Stacks

## ABDOMINAL STACK 1

Abdominal Stack 1 has five exercises. Each exercise will be done for 45 seconds with a 15-second break. Repeat once more to complete the 10-minute stack. You can either follow the steps below or use your phone to scan the QR code, and select  Abdominal Stack 1 from the menu to work out along with me. Wherever possible, an easier, modified version of the exercises is also available.

## 1. HUNDRED PREP 2

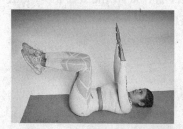 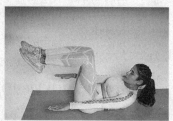

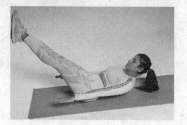

1. Lie supine on the mat with your legs in the table-top position (90/90). Make sure that your knees are directly over your hips and that your calves are parallel to the floor. Raise your arms to the ceiling.
2. Inhale to prepare, exhale to engage the abdominals and lift the head and upper body off the mat, simultaneously lowering the arm and extending the legs out at an angle that is diagonal to the mat.
3. Inhale and come back to the starting position in Step 1.
4. Repeat Steps 1 to 3 for 45 seconds.

**Make sure your lower back doesn't lift off the mat, and roll up only till the bottom tip of your shoulder blades.**

OR

**1A. MODIFICATION: HUNDRED PREP 1**

1. To modify, bend your knees and keep the feet hip-width apart on the mat. Follow Steps 2 and 3 above, and repeat for 45 seconds.

Break: 15 seconds.

**2.   ALL-FOURS HOVER HOLD**

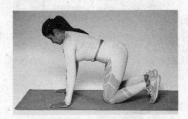 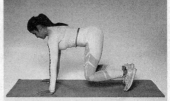

1. Start in the all-fours position with your wrists in line with your shoulders and knees in line with your hips. Press your hands into the mat and draw your shoulders down your back.

2.  Pressing into your hands and toes, lift your knees, hovering them slightly off the mat, while keeping your back neutral and chest open.
3.  Hold this position for 45 seconds.

OR
## 2A. MODIFICATION: ALL-FOURS UP AND DOWN

To modify, follow Steps 1 and 2, but instead of holding the position, alternate between lifting and resting your knees on the mat for 45 seconds. Make sure your back is neutral throughout the movement.

Break: 15 seconds.

## 3. CRISS CROSS

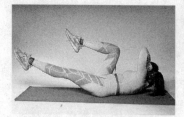 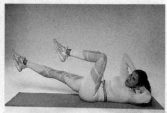

1.  Lie supine on the mat with your fingers interlaced behind your head.
2.  Lift your legs to the table-top position (90/90). Make sure that your knees are directly over your hips and that your calves are parallel to the floor. Lift your head and upper body off the mat.
3.  Bend one leg to bring the knee towards the chest as the other leg extends away from you at an angle diagonal to the mat.
4.  Rotate the torso as you switch legs.
5.  Repeat Steps 3 and 4 for 45 seconds.

**Keep your abdominals engaged and your elbows wide throughout the movement.**

OR
## 3A. MODIFICATION: ALTERNATE ELBOW TO KNEE

1. Lie supine on the mat with your knees bent and your feet hip-width apart.
2. Interlace your fingers and place them behind your head.
3. Lift one leg and bring the opposite shoulder towards the knee.
4. Place it down and repeat on the other side.
5. Keep switching sides for 45 seconds.

Break: 15 seconds.

## 4.  SIDE HOVER HOLD

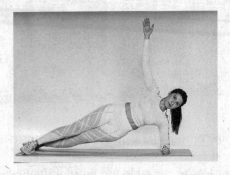

1. Lie on your side with your forearm on the mat. Press into the forearm to engage the lats.
2. Press into your feet to lift your hips up.
3. Extend your top hand towards the ceiling or place it on your waist, but not on the mat.
4. Hold this position for 20 seconds and switch sides for a total of 45 seconds.

OR

## 4A. MODIFICATION: FOREARM PLANK

**To get your body ready for the Side Hover Hold, you can start with the forearm plank.**

1. Place both your forearms on the mat, with your elbows in line with your shoulders and get into plank position. Press into the forearms to lift your shoulders, keeping your chest open and reaching your heels away from you as you stretch the legs. Engage your abdominals and squeeze your glutes. Your body should be in a straight line from your head to your heels.
2. Hold this position for 45 seconds.

Break: 15 seconds.

## 5. DIAMOND SIT-UP

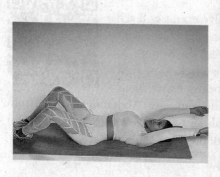 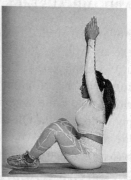

1. Lie supine on the mat with your legs in the diamond position such that your feet are together, and knees are apart.
2. Stretch your arms over your head.
3. Engage your abdominals and curl up into a seated position, extending your back at the top.
4. Roll your back down to the mat with control.
5. Repeat Steps 3 and 4 for 45 seconds.

OR
## 5A. MODIFICATION: DIAMOND CRUNCH

1.  Lie supine on the mat with your legs in a diamond, such that your feet are together, knees are apart.
2.  Stretch your arms overhead.
3.  Interlace your fingers and put your hands behind your head.
4.  Inhale and on the exhalation, curl your back up to do a crunch, and lower your back down on the mat. Make sure your elbows are wide.
5.  Repeat Step 4 for 45 seconds.

Break: 15 seconds.

*Repeat all five exercises to complete your 10-minute stack. Abdominal Stack 1 is done.*

## ABDOMINAL STACK 2

Abdominal Stack 2 has five exercises. Each exercise will be done for 45 seconds with a 15-second break. Repeat once more to complete the 10-minute stack. You can either follow the steps below or use your  phone to scan the QR code, and select Abdominal Stack 2 from the menu to work out along with me. Wherever possible, an easier, modified version of the exercises is also available.

1.  **DIAMOND CURLS**

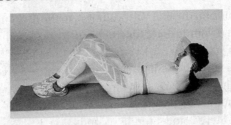

1. Lie supine on the mat with your legs in a diamond, such that your feet are together, knees are apart.
2. Interlace your fingers and place them behind your head.
3. Inhale to prepare and on the exhalation, curl up and engage your abdominals as you lower down.
4. Repeat Step 3 for 45 seconds.

**Don't touch your head to the mat, keep it hovering.**

Break: 15 seconds.

## 2. ROLLING LIKE A BALL

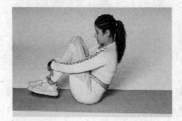 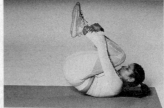

1. Sit on the mat with your knees bent, feet off the floor and arms around the shins, balancing between your sit bones and your tailbone.
2. Keep the abdominals engaged and draw your shoulders away from your ears and keep your elbows wide.
3. Curl your back and look into your bellybutton. Your head should be down and your chin should be tucked in.
4. Roll back to your shoulder blades and then roll up again.
5. Keep rolling back and up for 45 seconds, but don't touch your head to the mat.

OR

## 2A. MODIFICATION: ROLLING LIKE A BALL HOLD

1.  Follow Steps 1 to 3 and hold for 45 seconds. Keep drawing
    your belly button in towards the spine.

Break: 15 seconds.

## 3.  SINGLE LEG STRETCH

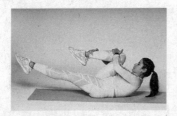 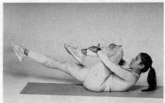

1.  Lie supine on the mat.
2.  Lift your legs to the table-top position (90/90). Make sure
    that your knees are directly over your hips and your calves
    are parallel to the floor.
3.  Hold the back of your thighs and come up to the tip of your
    shoulder blades.
4.  Pull one leg in and place the opposite hand on the knee, the
    same hand on the ankle and extend the other leg away from
    you. Keep your elbows wide, shoulders down your back and
    abdominals pulled in. Look at your knees and switch legs.
5.  Keep alternating legs for 45 seconds.

OR

## 3A. MODIFICATION: SINGLE LEG STRETCH WITH HEAD DOWN

Follow the steps in the exercise above, but keep your head down.

Break: 15 seconds.

## 4.   SEATED MERMAID TWIST

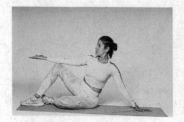 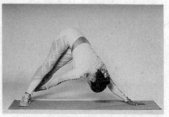

1.   Sit on the mat on the side of one hip with your knees bent. The top leg should be in front of the bottom leg, with your top knee towards the ceiling.
2.   Place the supporting hand diagonally on the mat, in scaption (slightly ahead of your shoulder). Press the palm into the mat to engage the lats and place the other hand on top of the bent knee with the palm facing up.
3.   Inhale and lift your hips up towards the ceiling. As your legs straighten, rotate and touch the back ankle. Press the supporting hand into the mat and keep the lats engaged.
4.   Lower the hips back to the starting position with control, and repeat.
5.   Repeat Steps 3 and 4 for 20 seconds and switch sides for a total of 45 seconds.

OR

## 4A. MODIFICATION: SIDE HOVER HOLD

To build strength on your sides for the Seated Mermaid Twist, follow the steps for the Side Hover Hold on page 148. Keep the bottom knee bent.

Break: 15 seconds.

## 5.  SINGLE STRAIGHT LEG STRETCH

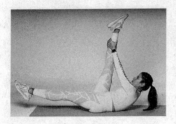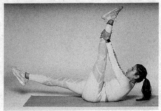

1.  Lie supine on the mat.
2.  Lift your head, chest and shoulders up till the tip of your shoulder blades and get your legs into the table-top position (90/90). Make sure that your knees are directly over your hips and that your calves are parallel to the floor.
3.  Lift one leg straight up towards the ceiling and keep the other leg straight out to just hover off the mat.
4.  'Walk' your hands up the top leg to wherever comfortable, keeping your elbows wide.
5.  Pulse that leg towards you and switch legs.
6.  Repeat Steps 3 to 5 for 45 seconds.

OR

## 5A. MODIFICATION: SINGLE STRAIGHT LEG STRETCH WITH HEAD DOWN

To modify, do the same exercise with your head down for 45 seconds.

Break: 15 seconds.

*Repeat all five exercises to complete your 10-minute stack. Abdominal Stack 2 is done.*

## ABDOMINAL STACK 3

Abdominal Stack 3 has five exercises. Each exercise will be done for 45 seconds with a 15-second break. Repeat once more to complete the 10-minute stack. You can either follow the steps below or use your

phone to scan the QR code, and select Abdominal Stack 3 from the menu to work out along with me. Wherever possible, an easier, modified version of the exercises is also available.

## 1.  PLANK TO PIKE

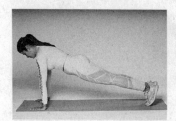 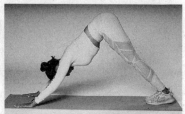

1.  Start in the plank position, with your wrists directly under your shoulders. Press into the mat so that your shoulders are away from it, keep your collar bone wide, engage your abdominals, and squeeze your glutes. Stretch your heels out away from you so that your legs are straight.
2.  From this position, pull your tailbone up towards the ceiling. Imagine someone has put a hook into your tailbone and is pulling you up.
3.  Return to the plank position.
4.  Repeat Steps 2 and 3 for 45 seconds.

OR

## 1A. MODIFICATION: ALL-FOURS TO PIKE

1.  Come into the all-fours position with your wrists in line with your shoulders and knees in line with your hips.

Keeping your back neutral, press into your hands to lift your shoulders away from the mat.

2. Curl your toes, straighten your knees and lift your hips up towards the ceiling to go into a pike.

3. Return to the all-fours position.

4. Repeat Steps 2 and 3 for 45 seconds.

Break: 15 seconds.

## 2. FOREARM PLANK HIP DIPS

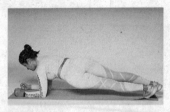 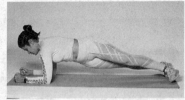

1. Place both your forearms on the mat such that your elbows are in line with your shoulders, and get into the plank position. Press into the forearms to lift your shoulders, keep your chest open, and stretch your heels away from you to lengthen the legs. Engage your abdominals and squeeze your glutes.

2. From this position, 'dip' your hips to one side, and then to the other, maintaining stability in the shoulders.

3. Keep alternating sides for 45 seconds.

OR
## 2A. MODIFICATION: FOREARM PLANK HOLD

1. Place both your forearms on the mat such that your elbows are in line with your shoulders, and get into the plank position. Press into the forearms to lift your shoulders, keep your chest open, and stretch your heels away from you to

lengthen the legs. Engage your abdominals and squeeze your glutes.
2.  Hold this position for 45 seconds.

Break: 15 seconds.

## 3.  X-MAN

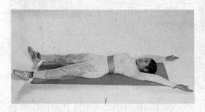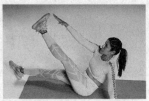

1.  Lie supine on the mat with your arms and legs stretched out away from each other, in an X.
2.  Pull your abdominals in, draw your ribs down towards your belly button and curl your pelvis slightly so that you don't hyperextend your lower back.
3.  From this position, sit up, simultaneously lifting one arm and the opposite leg, and touch the foot. Return to the starting position and repeat on the other side.
4.  Do this exercise in the flow for 45 seconds, and try to keep your arms and legs as straight as possible.

OR
## 3A. MODIFICATION: MODIFIED X-MAN

1.  Lie supine on the mat with your knees bent, feet flat on the mat, and your arms out in a V over your head.
2.  Lift one arm and extend the opposite leg to touch your toes.
3.  Place your foot back down and alternate with the opposite hand and leg. Keep alternating hands and legs for 45 seconds.

**In case you can't touch the toes, just touch the ankle or the furthest point on the leg.**

Break: 15 seconds.

## 4. CRAB TO REVERSE PLANK

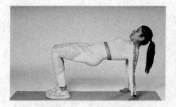 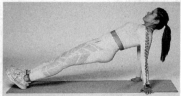

1. Sit on the mat with your knees bent, your arms behind you and your fingertips facing away from each other.
2. Draw your shoulders away from your ears.
3. Lift your hips off the mat and towards the ceiling looking straight ahead and pull your abdominals in.
4. From this position, straighten out one leg and then the other to get into a reverse plank.
5. Bend one knee and then the other to go back into a crab.
6. Repeat Steps 4 and 5 for 45 seconds.

OR
## 4A. MODIFICATION: CRAB LIFTS

1. Sit on the mat with your knees bent, your arms behind you and your fingertips facing away from each other.
2. Draw your shoulders away from your ears.
3. Lift your hips off the mat and towards the ceiling looking straight ahead and pull your abdominals in.
4. Fold at the hips to lower down towards the mat for a split second and lift up again.
5. Repeat Step 4 for 45 seconds.

Break: 15 seconds.

## 5.   REVERSE BENT KNEE CURL

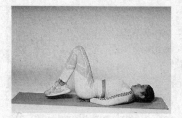 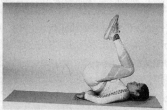

1.   Lie supine on the mat.
2.   Place your hands under your tailbone.
3.   Hover your feet off the mat while bending your knees.
4.   Look straight up at the ceiling while resting your head on the mat, and draw your shoulders down your back.
5.   Initiating with your abdominals, curl your pelvis to lift your hips off the mat, bringing your knees towards your face. Lower your hips down with control.
6.   Repeat Step 5 for 45 seconds.

OR

## 5A. MODIFICATION: ALTERNATE BENT KNEE LEG LIFTS

1.   Lie supine on the mat with your knees bent, feet flat on the mat and your arms out in a V by your side.
2.   Engage the abdominals and lift one foot off the floor keeping the hips stable. Place the foot back down on the mat.
3.   Alternate legs and repeat for 45 seconds.

Break: 15 seconds.

*Repeat all five exercises to complete your 10-minute stack. Abdominal Stack 3 is done.*

## ABDOMINAL STACK 4

Abdominal Stack 4 has five exercises. Each exercise will be done for 45 seconds with a 15-second break. Repeat once more to complete the 10-minute stack. You can either follow the steps below or use your phone to scan the QR code, and select  Abdominal Stack 4 from the menu to work out along with me. Wherever possible, an easier, modified version of the exercises is also available.

### 1. SIT-UP TO CRAB

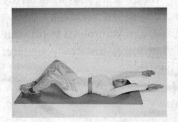 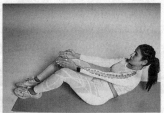

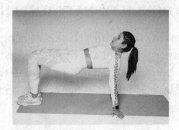

1. Lie supine on the mat with your legs in a diamond. Keep your feet together but knees apart.
2. Stretch your arms over your head.
3. Engage your abdominals and curl up into the seated position. Extend your back at the top and stretch your arms towards the ceiling.

4. Rotate your shoulders to place your hands on the mat behind you with your fingers pointing away from each other. Bend your knees and place your feet on the mat.
5. Lift your hips off the mat and towards the ceiling while looking straight ahead and pull your abdominals in to go into the crab position.
6. Lower back down, bring your legs into a diamond again with your hands in front, and roll back down on the mat with control.
7. Repeat Steps 2 to 6 for 45 seconds.

OR

**1A. MODIFICATION: CRUNCH TO BRIDGE**

1. Lie supine on the mat, with your knees bent and feet on the mat either together or hip-width apart. Keep your fingers interlaced behind your head.
2. Curl up and lift your head and shoulders off the mat and lower down to the mat.
3. Now lift your hips off the mat towards the ceiling to go into a bridge. Lower back down with control.
4. Repeat Steps 2 and 3 for 45 seconds.

Break: 15 seconds.

**2. SUPINE OPENINGS**

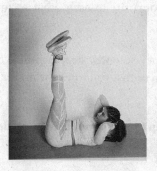
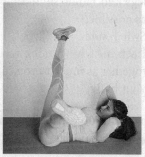

1.  Lie supine on the mat. Interlace your hands behind your head and lift your legs straight up towards the ceiling.
2.  Lift your head, chest and shoulders off the mat, and slide your shoulders down your back. Look straight ahead.
3.  Turn your feet out into a V with your heels together and toes apart. Point your feet and open your legs, flex your feet and close the legs.
4.  Repeat Step 3 for 45 seconds keeping your head, chest and shoulders lifted throughout the exercise.

Break: 15 seconds.

## 3.  RUSSIAN TWISTS

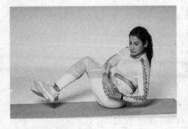 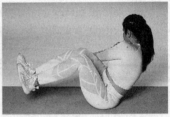

1.  Sit on the mat with your knees bent and lift your feet off the mat.
2.  Interlace your fingers in front of you.
3.  Move your hands to one side, and the legs to the other. The legs and hands should be opposite to each other as much as possible.
4.  Switch sides.
5.  Keep switching sides for 45 seconds, keeping the knees together as much as you can so that you work the midline of your body.

**Keep your abdominals pulled in towards your spine, and don't shrug your shoulders.**

OR

## 3A. MODIFICATION: MODIFIED RUSSIAN TWISTS

1.  Follow Steps 1 to 5 but don't lift your feet off the mat. Keep
    your feet planted on the mat, and keep switching sides for 45
    seconds.

Break: 15 seconds.

## 4.  PLANK TO PIKE WITH OPPOSITE ANKLE TAP

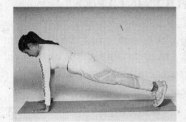
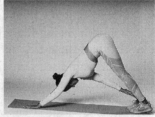
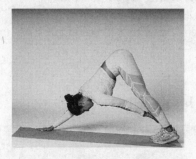

1.  Start in the plank position. Make sure your wrists are
    directly under your shoulders and press into the mat so
    that your shoulders are away from it. Keep your collarbone
    wide, engage your abdominals, and squeeze your glutes.
    Stretch your heels out away from you so that your legs
    are straight.

2.   From this position, pull your tailbone up towards the ceiling. Imagine someone has put a hook into your tailbone and is pulling you up.
3.   Tap one ankle with the opposite hand.
4.   Return to the plank position and tap the other ankle with the opposite hand.
5.   Alternate sides for 45 seconds.

OR

## 4A. MODIFICATION: ALL-FOURS INTO PIKE

1.   Come into the all-fours position with your wrists in line with your shoulders and knees in line with your hips. Keeping your back neutral, press into your hands to lift your shoulders away from the mat.
2.   Curl your toes, straighten your knees and lift your hips up towards the ceiling to go into a pike.
3.   Return to the all-fours position.
4.   Repeat Steps 2 and 3 for 45 seconds.

Break: 15 seconds.

## 5.   SEATED JACK KNIFE

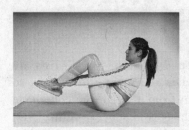 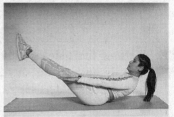

1.   Sit on the mat with your knees bent and lift your feet off the mat, balancing yourself between your tailbone and your sit bone. Keep your hands in front of you.

2. Extend both your legs diagonally to the mat, bend your knees, bring them towards your chest, and extend them out again.
3. Return to the starting position and repeat for 45 seconds. Alternate between reaching out and coming in.

OR

## 5A. MODIFICATION: MODIFIED SEATED JACK KNIFE

To modify this exercise, go down on your forearms, extend both your legs out and bring the alternate knee in towards your chest. Repeat the movement for 45 seconds.

Break: 15 seconds.

*Repeat all five exercises to complete your 10-minute stack. Abdominal Stack 4 is done.*

## ABDOMINAL STACK 5

Abdominal Stack 5 has five exercises. Each exercise will be done for 45 seconds with a 15-second break. Repeat once more to complete the 10-minute stack. You can either follow the steps below or use your phone to scan the QR code, and select  Abdominal Stack 5 from the menu to work out along with me. Wherever possible, an easier, modified version of the exercises is also available.

## 1. SIT-UP TO ALTERNATE HEEL TOUCH

1. Lie supine on the mat with your legs straight and arms over your head.

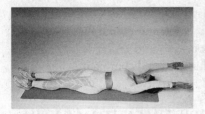 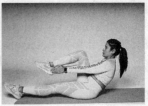

2. Inhale to prepare. On the exhalation, sit up and simultaneously bend one knee and touch the heel with both hands and lower back down with control.

3. Repeat, bending the other leg, and touching the other heel as you sit up. Make sure to draw your ribs down to your waist and draw your shoulders down your back. Don't shrug your shoulders.

4. Alternate sides for 45 seconds.

OR

## 1A. MODIFICATION: ALTERNATE HEEL TOUCH

1. Lie supine on the mat with your knees bent, feet on the floor and hands by your side.

2. Lift your head, chest and shoulders and laterally flex (bend) the spine to touch the heel and alternate sides.

3. Keep alternating sides for 45 seconds.

**Keep the head, chest and shoulders off the mat throughout the exercise.**

Break: 15 seconds.

## 2. SIDE KNEELING ELBOW TO KNEE

1. Kneel on the mat with your arms out to the sides in a T.

2. Lean over to one side until the hand touches the mat. Stretch the top leg and arm out and away from each other to create length and opposition in your sides.

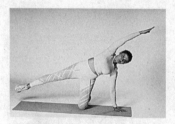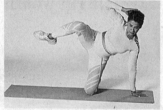

3. Press your supporting hand into the mat to activate your lats and draw your shoulders away from your ears.
4. Place your top hand behind your head and bring your top knee and elbow towards each other in lateral flexion.
5. Extend the top arm and leg away from each other to the starting position.
6. Repeat Steps 4 and 5 for 20 seconds and switch sides for a total of 45 seconds.

**When you reach back out, make sure to feel the opposition between your fingers and toes.**

OR

## 2A. MODIFICATION: SIDE LYING ELBOW TO KNEE ON FOREARM

1. Lie on your side and place the forearm on the mat in line with your shoulder. Press into the forearm to lift the torso off the mat. Flex at the hips to bring your legs slightly forward.
2. Place the top hand behind your head.
3. Laterally flex your spine, bending the top knee and flexing your upper body to bring the top elbow and knee together.
4. Extend the top arm and leg away from each other to the starting position.
5. Repeat Steps 3 and 4 for 20 seconds and switch sides for a total of 45 seconds.

Break: 15 seconds.

## 3.  AROUND THE WORLD

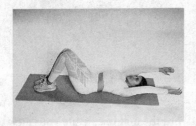
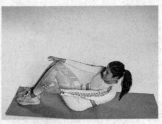

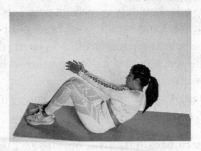

1.  Sit on the mat with your knees bent and feet on the mat. Interlace your fingers in front of you at shoulder level. Draw your shoulders down your back.
2.  Rotate your torso to the right and lower your back down to the mat on the right side. When your shoulder blades touch the mat, rotate your torso to the left. Keep your chin tucked in and come up on the left side to the seated position.
3.  Repeat Steps 1 and 2 on the other side.
4.  Continue alternating sides for 45 seconds.

OR
### 3A: MODIFICATION: CRUNCH

1.  Lie supine on the mat with your knees bent and feet on the mat.
2.  Interlace your fingers and place them behind your head.

3.  From this position, lift your head, chest and shoulders off the mat looking straight between your knees.
4.  Lower your head, chest and shoulders, and lift again.
5.  Keep lowering and lifting for 45 seconds.

Break: 15 seconds.

## 4.  BEAR FIRE FEET

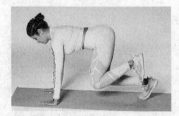 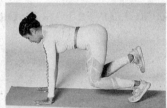

1.  Start in the all-fours position, with your wrists in line with your shoulders and knees in line with your hips.
2.  Press your hands into the mat and draw your shoulders down your back.
3.  Pressing into your hands and your toes, lift your knees, hovering them slightly off the mat while keeping your back neutral and chest open.
4.  Maintaining this position, lift the feet alternately off the mat in tempo (as fast as you can) for 45 seconds.

OR
## 4A. MODIFICATION: ALL-FOURS HOVER HOLD

1.  Start in the all-fours position with your wrists in line with your shoulders and knees in line with your hips.
2.  Press your hands into the mat and draw your shoulders down your back.

3. Pressing into your hands and your toes, lift your knees, hovering them slightly off the mat, while keeping your back neutral and chest open. Hold this position for 45 seconds.

**When you feel like you need a break, rest your knees and go back up only when you're ready.**

Break: 15 seconds.

## 5. ROLLOVER TO SCISSORS

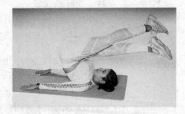 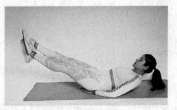

1. Lie supine on the mat with your legs in the table-top position (90/90). From this position, extend both legs diagonally to forty-five degrees.
2. Crisscross your legs, one on top of the other. Engage your abdominals, roll your back off the mat taking your legs behind you until parallel to the floor.
3. Return to the starting position with control, articulating your back on the mat as you continue to scissor your legs.
4. Go only as low as you can without hyperextending your back. Then, using your abdominals, lift your spine off to go into a rollover and come back into a scissors.
5. Alternate between the rollovers and the scissors for 45 seconds.

OR

## 5A. MODIFICATION: SCISSORS

1. Lie supine on the mat with your legs in the table-top position (90/90). Make sure that your knees are directly over your hips and your calves are parallel to the floor. Extend both legs diagonally to forty-five degrees and place your hands under your butt.
2. Crisscross your legs into a scissors, alternating legs for 45 seconds.
3. You can also lift your head up while crisscrossing your legs, to support your lower back.

Break: 15 seconds.

*Repeat all five exercises to complete your 10-minute stack. Abdominal Stack 5 is done.*

# 10-Minute Cardio Stacks

## CARDIO STACK 1

Cardio Stack 1 has five exercises. Each exercise will be done for 45 seconds with a 15-second break. Repeat once more to complete the 10-minute stack. You can either follow the steps below or use your phone to scan the QR code, and select

Cardio Stack 1 from the menu to work out along with me. Wherever possible, an easier, modified version of the exercises is also available.

## 1. BUTT KICK PUNCH

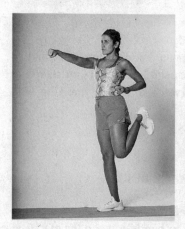 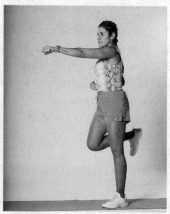

1. Stand upright with your feet hip-width apart.
2. Engage your abdominals.

3. From this position, kick your butt with your heel, and punch forward with the opposite hand simultaneously. You can also use the hand on the same side.
4. Switch hands and legs, and repeat Step 3.
5. Keep alternating hands and legs for 45 seconds.

Break: 15 seconds.

## 2.  HALF BURPEE

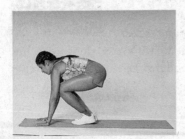 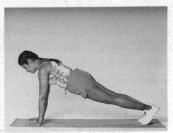

1. Stand upright at the front edge of your mat.
2. Bend at your knees to bring your hands down to the mat.
3. Jump back into a plank (see page 126 [Step 1] for reference of correct form), jump forward, and then jump up with your hands raised.
4. Repeat Step 3 for 45 seconds.

## OR
## 2A. MODIFICATION: STEP BACK BURPEE

1. Stand at the front edge of your mat.
2. Bend your knees to bring your hands down to the mat.
3. Step back into a plank one leg at a time (see page 126 [Step 1] for reference of correct form).
4. Step forward one leg at a time.

5. Stand upright, lifting your arms up towards the ceiling and heels off the mat at the same time.
6. Repeat Steps 1 to 5 for 45 seconds.

Break: 15 seconds.

## 3. GRAPEVINE WITH JUMP

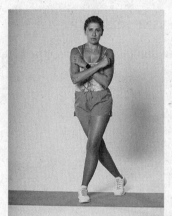 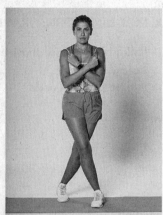

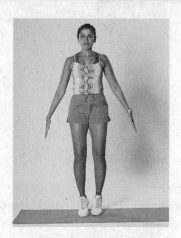

1.  Stand at the left side of your mat, facing forward.
2.  Take a big step to the right with the right foot and cross the left foot behind it.
3.  Take another step to the right with the right foot, bring the left foot to meet it and jump up.
4.  Alternate sides for 45 seconds.

OR

## 3A. MODIFICATION: GRAPEVINE HEELS UP

1.  Follow the exercise above but don't jump. Lift your heels up instead.
2.  Repeat for 45 seconds.

Break: 15 seconds.

## 4.  FRONT KICK

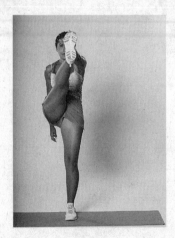

1.  Stand upright.
2.  Do a front kick with your right leg simultaneously punching forwards with your left hand.
3.  Repeat with the other arm and leg.
4.  Alternate for 45 seconds.

OR
## 4A. MODIFICATION: KNEE UP

1. Stand upright.
2. Bring your right knee up simultaneously bringing your left arm across.
3. Repeat on the other side.
4. Alternate for 45 seconds.

Break: 15 seconds.

## 5. TEMPO SIDE STEP

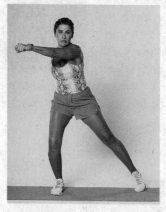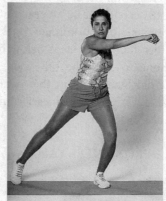

1. Stand upright.
2. Step out to the side with a hop and punch with the opposite hand. Repeat on the other side.
3. Keep alternating sides for 45 seconds.

OR
## 5A. MODIFICATION: SIDE STEP

1. Stand upright.
2. Step out to the side without a hop and punch with the opposite hand.

3. Repeat on the other side.
4. Keep alternating sides for 45 seconds.

Break: 15 seconds.

*Repeat all five exercises to complete your 10-minute stack.*
*Cardio Stack 1 is done.*

## CARDIO STACK 2

Cardio Stack 2 has five exercises. Each exercise will be done for 45 seconds with a 15-second break. Repeat once more to complete the 10-minute stack. You can either follow the steps below or use your phone to scan the QR code, and select
Cardio Stack 2 from the menu to work out along with me. Wherever possible, an easier, modified version of the exercises is also available.

### 1. FRONT HEEL TAP

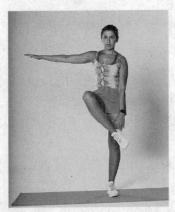 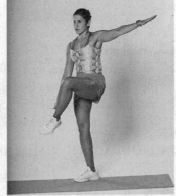

1. Stand upright with your feet slightly apart.
2. Stretch your arms out to the sides in a T.
3. Lift one leg up, bend your knee and tap your heel with the opposite hand.
4. Repeat with the other heel and hand.
5. Keep alternating sides for 45 seconds.

Break: 15 seconds.

## 2. SKATERS

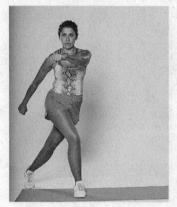 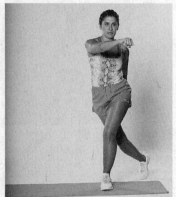

1. Stand upright with your feet shoulder-width apart.
2. Step out with your right leg and take your left leg diagonally behind it, hovering it off the floor.
3. Bring the left leg to step out to the other side and take your right leg diagonally behind it, hovering it off the floor.
4. Alternate sides with a hop to switch sides.
5. Add punching arms once you are comfortable with the movement.
6. Keep alternating sides for 45 seconds.

OR
## 2A. MODIFICATION: MODIFIED SKATERS

1.  Modify the exercise without the hop and hover.
2.  Repeat for 45 seconds.

Break: 15 seconds.

### 3.  REVERSE STEP BACK AND SIDE TAP

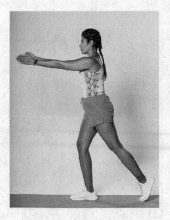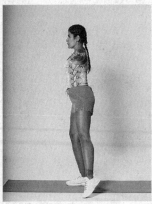

1.  Stand upright with your feet hip-width apart.
2.  Tap one leg to the back, then tap it to the side and then bring
    your legs back together.
3.  The supporting leg may bend slightly as you tap out to the
    side.
4.  Alternate with the other leg.
5.  Repeat for 45 seconds.

OR
## 3A. MODIFICATION: SIDE TAP

1.  Stand upright with your feet hip-width apart.

2. Take one leg out to the side, and back to the centre and then the other leg out to the side, and back to the centre.
3. Keep alternating legs for 45 seconds.

Break: 15 seconds.

## 4. SCISSORS

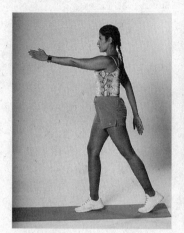 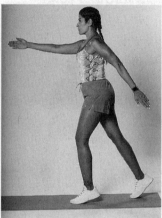

1. Stand upright with your feet hip-width apart.
2. With a jump, take one leg forward and the other leg back at the same time.
3. Jump and switch sides.
4. Keep alternating sides for 45 seconds.

OR

## 4A. MODIFICATION: STEP BACK

1. Stand upright with your feet hip-width apart.
2. Put your hands on your waist.

3.  Tap your legs back one after another as fast as you can for 45 seconds.
4.  As an option, you can also simultaneously use your hands to punch in the air.

Break: 15 seconds.

## 5.  360 SQUAT JUMP

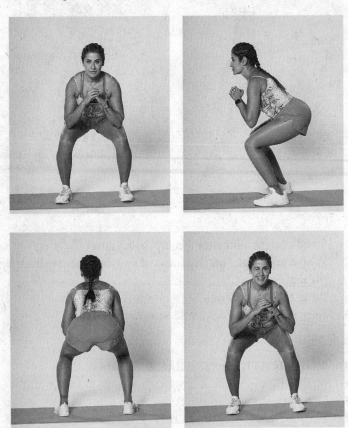

1.  Stand upright with your feet shoulder-width apart.
2.  Squat, using the form described on page 117.
3.  Maintaining the squat position, jump and rotate ninety degrees to the right. Keep rotating and jumping, maintaining the squat at a ninety degree turn until you're facing the front again.
4.  Switch directions to jump, squat, and rotate on the other side.
5.  Keep your back neutral throughout the exercise.
6.  Repeat for 45 seconds, switching directions after four rotating ninety-degree jump squats.

OR
## 5A. MODIFICATION: SQUATS

1.  Stand with your feet shoulder-width apart.
2.  Squat, using the form described on page 117, and extend the knees to come back up to the starting position.
3.  Repeat Step 2 for 45 seconds.

Break: 15 seconds.

*Repeat all five exercises to complete your 10-minute stack.*
*Cardio Stack 2 is done.*

## CARDIO STACK 3

Cardio Stack 3 has five exercises. Each exercise will be done for 45 seconds with a 15-second break. Repeat once more to complete the 10-minute stack. You can either follow the steps below or use your  phone to scan the QR code, and select Cardio Stack 3 from the menu to work out along with me. Wherever possible, an easier, modified version of the exercises is also available.

## 1. POGO JUMPS

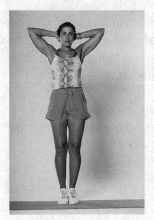 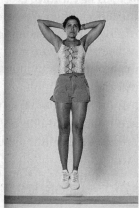

1. Stand upright with your feet hip-width apart.
2. Interlace your fingers and place your hands behind your head.
3. Keep your elbows wide and engage your abdominals.
4. Jump in place for 45 seconds.

**To make the exercise more challenging, keep your feet together. Maintain the upright position throughout the jump.**

OR
## 1A. MODIFICATION: HEEL LIFTS

1. To modify, lift your heels instead of jumping.
2. Repeat for 45 seconds.

Break: 15 seconds.

## 2.  SIDE STEP HOP

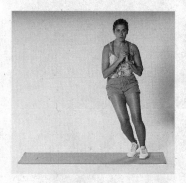 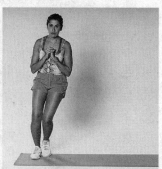

1.  Stand upright on the left side of your mat with your feet together.
2.  Take a long leap sideways to the right and bring the left foot to meet it.
3.  Take a long leap to the left and bring the right foot to meet it.
4.  Leap from side to side for 45 seconds.

OR
## 2A. MODIFICATION: SIDE STEP

1.  Stand upright on the side of your mat with your feet together.
2.  Take a long step sideways to the right and bring the left leg together and repeat on the other side. Step from side to side for 45 seconds.
3.  You can clasp your hands together in front of your chest.

Break: 15 seconds.

## 3.  HIGH KNEE PULLS

1.  Stand upright with your feet slightly apart.
2.  Raise your hands to the ceiling.

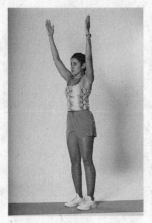 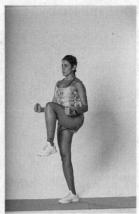

3. As you bring your hands down, get one knee to your chest.
4. Raise your hands up and alternate with the other knee.
5. Keep alternating knees for 45 seconds.

Break: 15 seconds.

## 4. JUMPING JACKS

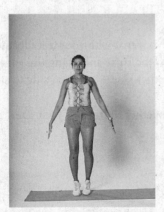 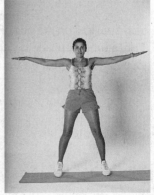

1. Stand upright with your feet slightly apart.
2. Split your legs and arms to go into a jack.
3. Jump back to the starting position.
4. Repeat Steps 2 and 3 for 45 seconds.

OR

## 4A. MODIFICATION: MODIFIED JUMPING JACKS

1. Stand upright with your feet slightly apart.
2. Step out to the side, one leg at a time.
3. Keep alternating legs for 45 seconds.

**Your arms can be on your waist or out to the side in a T as you step out.**

Break: 15 seconds.

## 5. POP SQUATS

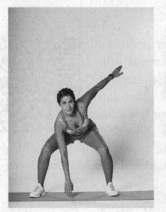 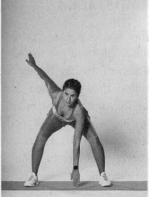

1. Stand upright with your feet slightly apart.
2. Jump out to go into a deep squat and touch the floor with one hand. The other hand must be pointing straight towards the ceiling.

3.  Jump back to the starting position and go into a deep squat bringing the other hand to touch the floor. Make sure the other hand is pointing straight towards the ceiling.
4.  Repeat Steps 2 and 3 for 45 seconds.

OR
## 5A. MODIFICATION: SUMO SQUATS

1.  Stand upright with feet wide and toes turned out.
2.  Go into a squat and come back up.
3.  Repeat this movement for 45 seconds.

Break: 15 seconds.

*Repeat all five exercises to complete your 10-minute stack.*
*Cardio Stack 3 is done.*

## CARDIO STACK 4

Cardio Stack 4 has five exercises. Each exercise will be done for 45 seconds with a 15-second break. Repeat once more to complete the 10-minute stack. You can either follow the steps below or use your phone to scan the QR code, and select  Cardio Stack 4 from the menu to work out along with me. Wherever possible, an easier, modified version of the exercises is also available.

### 1. STANDING HIP CIRCLES

1.  Stand upright with your feet hip-width apart.
2.  Put your hands on your waist.

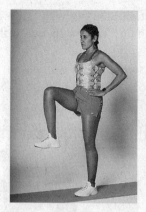 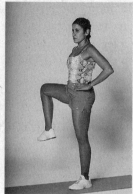

3. Lift one knee, circle it around and bring it back.
4. Alternate with the other knee.
5. Keep alternating knees for 45 seconds.

**Make sure you lift your knee as high as you can, keeping your lower back neutral.**

Break: 15 seconds.

## 2.   MODIFIED PLANK JACKS

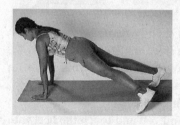 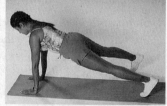

1. Start in the plank position. Make sure your wrists are directly under your shoulders and press into the mat so that your shoulders are away from it. Keep your collar bone wide, engage your abdominals, and squeeze your glutes. Reach your heels out away from you so that your legs are straight.

2.  Maintaining the plank position, step out with one leg and return to the starting position. Then step out with the other leg.
3.  Keep alternating legs for 45 seconds.

Break: 15 seconds.

### 3.   ALTERNATE HEEL TOUCH FRONT AND BACK

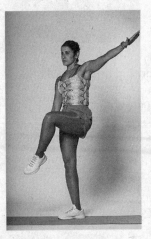 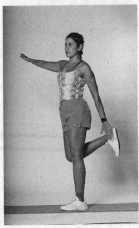

1.  Stand upright with your feet slightly apart.
2.  Stretch your arms out to the sides in a T.
3.  Lift the right leg up, bend your knee and tap your heel with the opposite hand.
4.  Repeat with the left leg and opposite hand.
5.  Now, take the right leg behind you and touch the heel with the opposite hand.
6.  Repeat with the left leg and opposite hand.
7.  Add a hop as you tap your heels.
8.  Keep alternating with the front and back heel taps for 45 seconds.

OR

## 3A. MODIFICATION: ALTERNATE HEEL TOUCH FRONT AND BACK (NO JUMPING)

1. Do the exercise without the hop.
2. Continue for 45 seconds.

Break: 15 seconds.

## 4. MOUNTAIN CLIMBERS

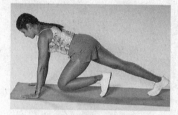 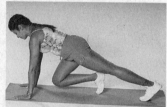

1. Start in the plank position. Make sure your wrists are directly under your shoulders and press into the mat so that your shoulders are away from it. Keep your collar bone wide, engage your abdominals, and squeeze your glutes. Reach your heels out away from you so that your legs are straight.
2. Maintaining the plank, bring one knee to the chest, hovering the foot off the mat and then switch with the other leg.
3. Keep alternating legs for 45 seconds.

**Do it in tempo to increase the intensity, keeping your torso stable.**

OR

## 4A. MODIFICATION: MODIFIED MOUNTAIN CLIMBERS

1. Start in the plank position, as mentioned above.

2.  Maintaining the plank, bring one knee to the chest, tapping the foot on the mat.
3.  Alternate with the other knee, tapping the front of the foot on the mat again. Don't forget to maintain stability in the torso.
4.  Keep alternating feet for 45 seconds.

Break: 15 seconds.

## 5. CROSS STEP JACK

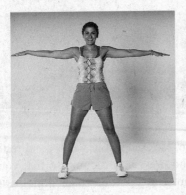 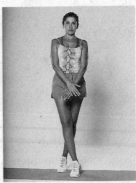

1.  Stand upright with your feet apart and your arms in a T.
2.  Jump and cross one leg in front of the other, crossing your hands in front of your hips.
3.  Jump out to go back to the starting position.
4.  Follow Step 2, except cross the other leg. Jump out to go back to the starting position.
5.  Repeat Steps 1 to 4 for 45 seconds, alternating legs.

OR
## 5A. MODIFICATION: STEP OUT

1.  Stand upright.
2.  Step out to the side with one leg and get back to the centre.

3. Repeat on the other side.
4. Keep alternating sides for 45 seconds.

Break: 15 seconds.

*Repeat all five exercises to complete your 10-minute stack.*
*Cardio Stack 4 is done.*

## CARDIO STACK 5

Cardio Stack 5 has five exercises. Each exercise will be done for 45 seconds with a 15-second break. Repeat once more to complete the 10-minute stack. You can either follow the steps below or use your phone to scan the QR code, and select  Cardio Stack 5 from the menu to work out along with me. Wherever possible, an easier, modified version of the exercises is also available.

### 1. REVERSE LUNGE WITH KNEE UP

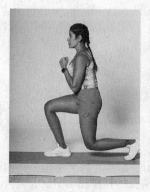
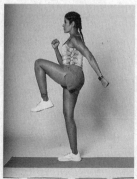

1. Stand upright with your feet hip-width apart.
2. Step back with your right foot and lower it down towards the floor as you bend the left knee.

3.   Your left thigh will be almost parallel to the floor.
4.   Pressing your left heel into the floor, bring your right leg forwards into a knee up. Repeat.
5.   Repeat for 20 seconds and switch sides for a total of 45 seconds.

OR

## 1A. MODIFICATION: ALTERNATE REVERSE LUNGE

1.   Stand upright with your feet hip-width apart.
2.   Step back with your right foot and lower it down towards the floor as you bend the left knee.
3.   Your left thigh will be almost parallel to the floor.
4.   Pressing your left heel into the floor, return to the standing position by bringing your right leg forward.
5.   Alternate legs, stepping back with the left foot.
6.   Keep alternating legs for 45 seconds.

Break: 15 seconds.

## 2.   HIGH PLANK ROLL

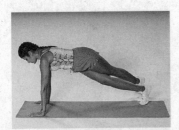 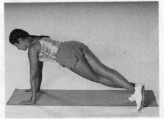

1.   Start in the plank position. Make sure your wrists are directly under your shoulders. Press into the mat so that your shoulders are away from it, keep your collar bone wide,

engage your abdominals, and squeeze your glutes. Stretch your heels out away from you so that your legs are straight.

2. From this position, cross one leg over the other without bending the bottom leg. Tap your foot to the floor, and come back to the plank position. Do the same with the other leg.

3. Keep your shoulders stable as your lower body rotates.

4. Alternate legs for 45 seconds.

OR

## 2A. MODIFICATION: ALL-FOURS ROLL

1. Come into the all-fours position with your wrists in line with your shoulders and knees in line with your hips. Keeping your back neutral, press into your hands to lift your shoulders away from the mat.

2. From this position, extend one leg and cross it over the other, tap your foot to the floor, and come back to the all-fours position. Do the same with the other leg.

3. Keep your shoulders stable as your lower body moves.

4. Alternate legs for 45 seconds.

Break: 15 seconds.

## 3. SQUAT STEP OUT

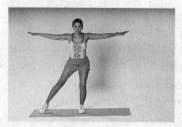
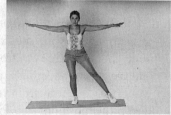

1. Stand upright with your feet hip-width apart, flex at the hips and go into a squat. Extend your arms out into a T.

2. From this position, extend one leg out laterally and tap on the mat. Return to the centre and alternate with the other leg.
3. Keep alternating legs for 45 seconds.
4. Increase the pace to increase the intensity.

Break: 15 seconds.

## 4. MODIFIED SQUAT THRUST

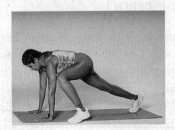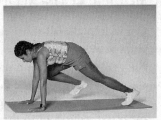

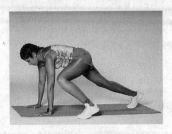

1. Start in the plank position, making sure your wrists are directly under your shoulders. Press into the mat so that your shoulders are away from it, keep your collar bone wide, engage your abdominals, and squeeze your glutes. Reach your heels out away from you so that your legs are straight.
2. From this position, step forward with your right foot and place it next to your right hand.
3. Then bring your left leg forward and place it next to your left hand.

4.  Return to the plank position, one leg at a time.
5.  Alternate legs for 45 seconds.

**Do this at a good pace for a cardio workout.**

## 4A. MODIFICATION: MODIFIED MOUNTAIN CLIMBER

1.  Start in a plank following Step 1 above.
2.  Bring one leg forward, tap the foot on the mat and take it back to the starting position. Do the same with the other leg.
3.  Keep alternating legs for 45 seconds.

Break: 15 seconds.

## 5.  SIDE STEP WITH FRONT AND LATERAL RAISE

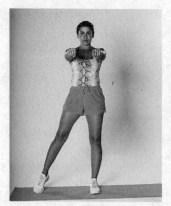 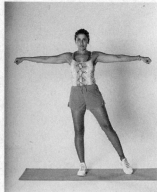

1.  Stand upright with your arms by your side.
2.  Tap out to the side with one leg as you lift both arms to the front at shoulder level.
3.  Lower your arms bringing your leg back to the centre.
4.  Tap the other leg out as you lift both arms to a T.

5. Bring your arms and legs back to the centre.
6. Repeat Steps 2 to 5 for 45 seconds.

Break: 15 seconds.

*Repeat all five exercises to complete your 10-minute stack.*
*Cardio Stack 5 is done.*

10-Minute Full Body Stacks

## FULL BODY STACK 1

Full Body Stack 1 has five exercises. Each exercise will be done for 45 seconds with a 15-second break. Repeat once more to complete the 10-minute stack. You can either follow the steps below or use your phone to scan the QR code, and select  Full Body Stack 1 from the menu to work out along with me. Wherever possible, an easier, modified version of the exercises is also available.

## 1. WIDE SQUAT PLANK WITH MIDAS TOUCH

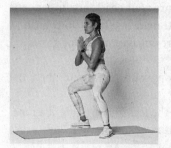
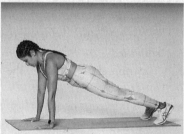
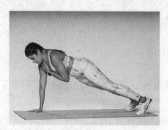

1.  Stand upright with your feet in a wide turned-out position. Flex at the hips to squat.
2.  Place your hands on the mat, and jump back to go into a plank. Make sure your wrists are under your shoulders, your body is in a straight line from your head to your heels, your abdominals are engaged and your glutes are squeezed.
3.  Tap one shoulder with the opposite hand, and then the other.
4.  Press into your hands to jump forward, landing wide with your feet, and lift your torso into a wide squat.
5.  Repeat Steps 2 to 4 for 45 seconds.

OR

### 1A. MODIFICATION: WIDE SQUAT WALK OUT TO PLANK

1.  Stand upright with your feet in a wide turned-out position. Flex at the hips to squat.
2.  Place your hands on the mat, step back with one leg, then the other into a plank. Make sure your wrists are under your shoulders, your body is in a straight line from your head to your heels, your abdominals are engaged and your glutes are squeezed.
3.  Tap one shoulder with the opposite hand, and then the other.
4.  Press into your hands to bring the legs forward one at a time, keeping your feet wide, and lift your torso into a wide squat and stand up.
5.  Repeat Steps 2 to 4 for 45 seconds.

Break: 15 seconds.

### 2.  CRAB ALTERNATE HAND TO FOOT TAP

1.  Sit on the mat with your knees bent and your arms behind you with your fingertips facing away from each other.

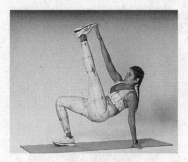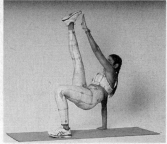

2.  Draw your shoulders away from your ears.
3.  As you lift your hips off the mat towards the ceiling, extend one leg and the opposite hand towards each other, and try to tap the leg with your hand.
4.  Fold at the hips to lower down towards the mat to the starting position for a split second and lift up again, this time extending the other leg and hand towards each other, and again try to tap the leg with your hand.
5.  Alternate legs and hands for 45 seconds.

OR

## 2A. MODIFICATION: CRAB BRIDGE

1.  Sit on the mat with your knees bent and your arms behind you with your fingertips facing away from each other.
2.  Draw your shoulders away from your ears.
3.  Lift your hips off the mat towards the ceiling looking straight ahead and pulling your abdominals in.
4.  Fold at the hips to lower down towards the mat for a split second and lift up again.
5.  Repeat Steps 3 and 4 for 45 seconds.

Break: 15 seconds.

## 3.   INCHWORM TO ALTERNATE LUNGE AND ROTATE

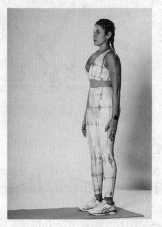
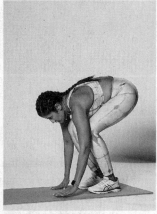

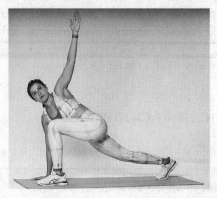

1.   Stand upright with your feet hip-width apart.
2.   Inhale, take your arms up.
3.   Exhale and roll down towards the floor, bending your knees, and place your hands on the mat.
4.   From this position, 'walk' forward with your hands into a plank in four counts.

5.  Bring your right leg forward to place it on the mat between your hands, simultaneously taking the right arm up towards the ceiling in rotation.
6.  Bring the leg back to go into a plank and bending your knees, 'walk' your hands back towards your feet in four counts and stand up.
7.  Repeat Steps 1 to 6, lunging this time with the left leg and rotate taking the left arm up towards the ceiling.
8.  Alternate sides for 45 seconds.

OR

**3A. MODIFICATION: INCHWORM TO PLANK**

1.  Stand upright with your feet hip-width apart.
2.  Inhale, take your arms up.
3.  Exhale and roll down towards the floor, bending your knees, and place your hands on the mat.
4.  From this position, 'walk' forward with your hands into a plank in four counts. Make sure your wrists are under your shoulders, your body is in a straight line from your head to your heels, your abdominals are engaged and your glutes are squeezed.
5.  Bend your knees, and 'walk' your hands back towards your feet.
6.  Roll back up.
7.  Repeat Steps 1 to 6 for 45 seconds.

Break: 15 seconds.

**4.  OPPOSITE ELBOW TO KNEE AND STRAIGHT KICK**

1.  Stand upright with your hands behind your head.
2.  Lift your right knee and contract your torso to bring your left elbow towards it.

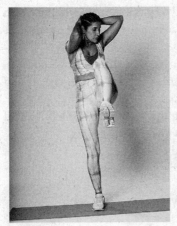 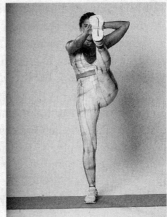

3.  Lower the leg down, extending the torso.
4.  Kick the right leg up and extending the left hand in front, touch the right foot.
5.  Repeat Steps 1 to 4 with the opposite side.
6.  Keep alternating sides for 45 seconds.

OR

## 4A. MODIFICATION: OPPOSITE ELBOW TO KNEE ALTERNATE SIDES

1.  Stand upright with your hands behind your head.
2.  Lift your right knee and contract your torso to bring your left elbow towards it.
3.  Lower the leg down, extending the torso.
4.  Alternate with the other elbow and knee.
5.  Keep alternating sides for 45 seconds.

Break: 15 seconds.

## 5.   INVISIBLE BALL SLAMS

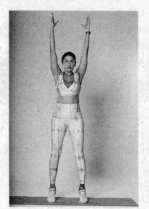 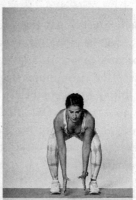

1.  Stand upright with your feet shoulder-width apart.
2.  Imagine you have a ball in your hands and that you're holding the ball in front of your chest.
3.  From this position, raise your arms and heels to go up on the balls of your feet and, flexing at your hips, 'slam' the ball down. Your heels will automatically go back down.
4.  Go up again, and slam. Repeat for 45 seconds.

OR

## 5A. MODIFICATION: INVISIBLE BALL SLAMS WITH NO HEEL LIFT

1.  Stand upright with your feet shoulder-width apart.
2.  Imagine you have a ball in your hands, and that you're holding the ball in front of your chest.
3.  From this position, raise your arms up and, flexing at your hips, 'slam' the ball down. Don't lift your heels up.
4.  Go up again, and slam. Repeat for 45 seconds.

Break: 15 seconds.

*Repeat all five exercises to complete your 10-minute stack.*
*Full Body Stack 1 is done.*

# FULL BODY STACK 2

Full Body Stack 2 has five exercises. Each exercise will be done for 45 seconds with a 15-second break. Repeat once more to complete the 10-minute stack. You can either follow the steps below or use your phone to scan the QR code, and select  Full Body Stack 2 from the menu to work out along with me. Wherever possible, an easier, modified version of the exercises is also available.

## 1. KNEELING SQUATS

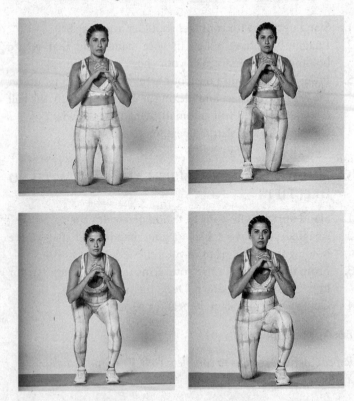

1. Stand upright with your feet hip-width apart.
2. Kneel down on the mat one knee at a time.
3. Come back up to a squat position (see form on page 117). You can also take breaks from the squat by standing upright if it is too challenging to maintain the squat position.
4. Repeat on the same side or alternate legs for 45 seconds.

OR

**1A. MODIFICATION: ALTERNATE REVERSE LUNGE**

1. Stand upright with your feet hip-width apart.
2. Step back with your right foot, lowering the knee towards the mat as you simultaneously bend the left knee.
3. Your left thigh should be almost parallel to the floor.
4. Pressing your left heel into the floor, return to the standing position by bringing your right leg forward.
5. Alternate legs, stepping back with the left foot this time.
6. Keep alternating legs for 45 seconds.

Break: 15 seconds.

**2. RENEGADE ROW**

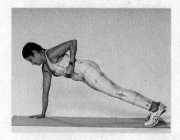
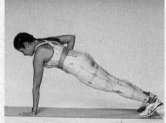

1. Start in the plank position, making sure your wrists are directly under your shoulders. Press into the mat so that

your shoulders are away from it, keep your collar bone wide, engage your abdominals, and squeeze your glutes. Reach your heels out and away from you so that your legs are straight.

2. From this position, imagine you now have a dumbbell in both hands. Bend at one elbow to 'row' the dumbbell towards your waist.

3. Place your hand back down, and repeat with the other hand.

4. Keep alternating hands for 45 seconds. Make sure to keep your body stable and try not to shift it too much to one side.

OR

## 2A. MODIFICATION: ALL-FOURS RENEGADE ROW

1. Come into the all-fours position with wrists in line with your shoulders and knees in line with your hips. Keeping your back neutral, press into your hands to lift your shoulders away from the mat.

2. Follow Steps 2 to 4 above.

Break: 15 seconds.

## 3. ALTERNATE ELBOW TO KNEE AND STARJACK

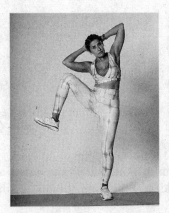
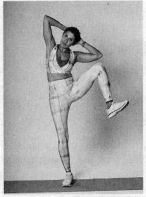

1. Stand upright with your feet hip-width apart.
2. Interlace your fingers and place them behind your head. Keep your elbows wide.
3. Side bend at the waist to the right and laterally bring your right knee up towards your right elbow.
4. Repeat on the left side.
5. Bring both hands down to the side and jump taking your legs wide and arms in a T.
6. Return to the starting position.
7. Repeat Steps 1 to 6 for 45 seconds.

Break: 15 seconds.

## 4. FOREARM PLANK TO ROTATION

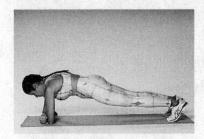 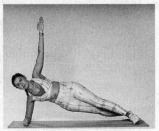

1. Start in a forearm plank. Make sure that your elbows are under your shoulders and your body is in a straight line from your head to your heels. Engage your abdominals, and squeeze your glutes. Reach your heels away from you so that your knees are straight.
2. Bring your right fist towards your left elbow and your left fist towards your right elbow, making sure your forearms are parallel to each other.
3. From this position rotate on the left side taking your right arm towards the ceiling.

4. Return to the centre and repeat on the other side.
5. Alternate sides for 45 seconds.

OR
## 4A. MODIFICATION: FOREARM PLANK HOLD

1. Follow Step 1 above to get into a forearm plank.
2. Hold for 45 seconds.

Break: 15 seconds.

## 5. SUPERMAN

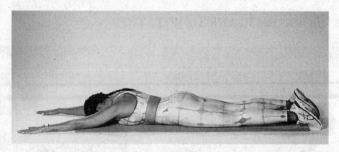

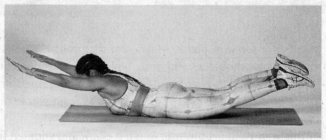

1. Lie prone on your stomach. Your arms and legs should be reaching away from each other. Think of your toes and fingertips being in opposition, pulling away from each other.

2.   Engage your abdominals, squeeze your glutes.
3.   Draw your shoulders away from your ear.
4.   Float your arms and legs up simultaneously, keeping your torso stable.
5.   Float your head up keeping your ears between your arms.
6.   Lower down with control.
7.   Repeat Steps 4 to 6 for 45 seconds.

OR

## 5A. MODIFICATION: OPPOSITE ARM AND LEG LIFT

1.   Lie prone on the mat, with your arms and legs reaching out in opposite directions.
2.   Pull your abdominals away from the mat, and squeeze your glutes.
3.   From this position, slide your shoulders down your back, lift the opposite arm and leg off the mat and then lower them back down.
4.   Lift the other arm and leg and lower back down.
5.   Alternate arms and legs for 45 seconds.

**As you lift, think that the energy is going out from the two ends of your body.**

Break: 15 seconds.

*Repeat all five exercises to complete your 10-minute stack.*
*Full Body Stack 2 is done.*

## FULL BODY STACK 3

Full Body Stack 3 has five exercises. Each exercise will be done for 45 seconds with a 15-second break. Repeat once more to complete the 10-minute stack. You can either follow the steps below or use your phone to scan the QR code, and select Full Body Stack

3 from the menu to work out along with me. Wherever possible, an easier, modified version of the exercises is also available.

### 1.  SIDE LYING CLAMS WITH HIP LIFT

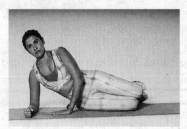 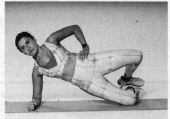

1.  Lie on your side on your forearm, elbows in line with your shoulders.
2.  Press your forearm into the mat to engage your lats, and slide your shoulder away from your ear.
3.  Keeping your knees in line with your hips, fold them at a ninety-degree angle placing your feet behind you.
4.  Your other hand can be either on the mat or on your waist.
5.  Making sure your hips are stacked on top of each other, and keeping your feet together, lift the top knee and the hips off the floor, and then lower both and lift again, without disturbing the alignment of the hips and shoulders—you should feel this exercise in your glutes.
6.  Repeat for 20 seconds and switch sides for a total of 45 seconds.

OR
## 1A. MODIFICATION: SIDE LYING CLAMS

1. To modify this exercise, change the starting position by bringing your knees forward and keeping your heels in line with your glutes. Follow the rest of the exercise as given, but don't lift the hips.
2. Repeat for 20 seconds and switch sides for a total of 45 seconds.

Break: 15 seconds.

## 2. SEATED TRICEPS TO FOREARMS

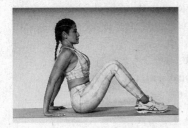 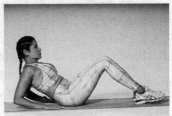

1. Sit on your mat with your knees bent and your hands behind you, fingers pointing towards your toes.
2. Press into the mat and bring your shoulders away from your ears.
3. From this position, bend your elbows to come on to your forearms, and then extend your elbows to come back to the starting position.
4. Remember to lower yourself down with control.
5. Repeat Step 3 for 45 seconds.

Break: 15 seconds.

### 3.  SINGLE LEG HAMSTRING CURLS

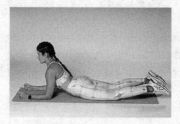 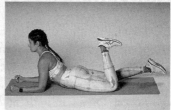

1.  Lie prone on the mat.
2.  Press into the mat to come up on to your forearms, your pelvis on the mat.
3.  Press into your forearms to move your shoulders away from your ears, and slide them down your back. Engage your abdominals and squeeze your glutes hovering your legs off the floor.
4.  Bend one knee and pulse the heel twice.
5.  Extend the leg back and repeat with the other leg.
6.  Alternate legs for 45 seconds.

Break: 15 seconds.

### 4.  SINGLE LEG DEADLIFTS

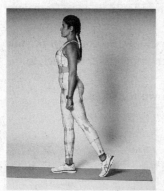 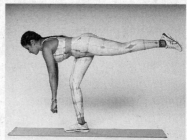

1. Stand upright with your feet hip-width apart.
2. Hinge at the hips to take your torso towards the floor, keeping your back neutral, simultaneously lifting one leg straight back.
3. The standing leg will bend slightly as you hinge and the arms will reach towards the floor. Engage your glutes to extend back up to the starting position.
4. Repeat Steps 1 to 3 for about 20 seconds and switch sides for a total of 45 seconds.

OR
**4A. MODIFICATION: DOUBLE LEG DEADLIFTS**

1. Stand upright with your feet hip-width apart.
2. Hinge at the hips, keep your back flat, chest open, and lower your torso towards the floor.
3. Keep your knees slightly bent as you lower and engage your core.
4. Engage your glutes to extend back up to the starting position.
5. Repeat Steps 1 to 4 for 45 seconds.

Break: 15 seconds.

**5. BEAR JACKS**

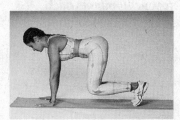 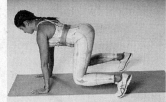

1.  Start in an all-fours position, wrists in line with your shoulders, knees in line with your hips.
2.  Press your hands into the mat and draw your shoulders down your back.
3.  Pressing into your hands and your toes, lift your knees, hovering them slightly off the mat, while keeping your back neutral and chest open.
4.  Keeping the upper body stable, separate at your knees taking your feet into a jack and back together.
5.  Repeat Step 4 for 45 seconds.

OR
## 5A. MODIFICATION: ALL-FOURS HOVER

1.  Start in an all-fours position, wrists in line with your shoulders, knees in line with your hips.
2.  Press your hands into the mat and draw your shoulders down your back.
3.  Pressing into your hands and your toes, lift your knees, hovering them slightly off the mat, while keeping your back neutral and chest open.
4.  Hold this position for 45 seconds.

Break: 15 seconds.

*Repeat all five exercises to complete your 10-minute stack.*
*Full Body Stack 3 is done.*

## FULL BODY STACK 4

Full Body Stack 4 has five exercises. Each exercise will be done for 45 seconds with a 15-second break. Repeat once more to complete the 10-minute stack. You can either follow the steps below or use your phone to scan the QR code, and select  Full Body Stack 4 from the menu to work out along with me. Wherever possible, an easier, modified version of the exercises is also available.

### 1. SQUAT TO *RELEVÉ*

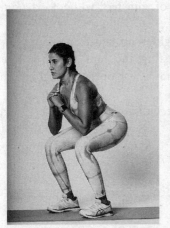 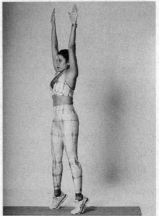

1. Stand upright with your feet shoulder-width apart, toes slightly turned out.
2. Engage your abdominals, flex at the hips, push them back and lower down as if sitting on an invisible chair. Let your knees follow the direction of your feet, without extending them over your toes.

3.  Extend your legs and straighten up and simultaneously lift your heels to go up on the balls of your feet into a *relevé*. Keep your back neutral and your chest open throughout the movement.
4.  Repeat Steps 1 to 3 for 45 seconds.

OR

## 1A. MODIFICATION: WIDE SQUAT

1.  Stand upright with your feet slightly wider than shoulder-width apart, toes slightly turned out.
2.  Engage your abdominals, flex at the hips, push them back and lower down as if sitting on an invisible chair. Let your knees follow the direction of your feet, without extending them over your toes.
3.  Extend your legs and straighten up, squeezing your glutes at the top, without thrusting the hips forward. Keep your back neutral and your chest open throughout the movement.
4.  Repeat Steps 1 to 3 for 45 seconds.

Break: 15 seconds.

## 2.  DIAMOND PUSH-UP

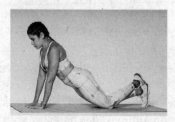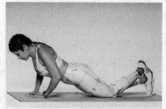

1.  Place your hands on the mat and touch your middle fingers, index fingers and thumbs to each other to form a diamond.

2. Extend your legs to come into a plank, making sure your wrists are under your shoulders, your body is in a straight line from your head to your heels, your abdominals are engaged and your glutes are squeezed.
3. Bend your arms at the elbow and lower your body towards the mat in a straight line, and use your triceps to extend your elbows and push yourself back up.
4. Repeat Step 3 for 45 seconds.

OR
## 2A. MODIFICATION: DIAMOND PUSH-UP ON KNEES

1. Follow Step 1 above.
2. Get into a modified plank with your knees on the mat. Make sure your wrists are under your shoulders, your body is in a straight line from your head to your knees, your abdominals are engaged and your glutes are squeezed.
3. Bend your arms at the elbow to lower your body towards the mat in a straight line. Use your triceps to extend your elbows and push yourself back up.
4. Repeat Step 3 for 45 seconds.

Break: 15 seconds.

## 3. DEAD BUG

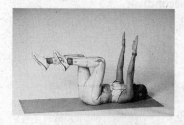 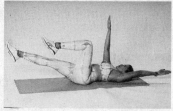

1. Lie supine on your back with your hands straight up towards the ceiling, but in line with your shoulders.

2. Lift your feet off the mat, and bend your legs at the knees at a ninety-degree angle to reach the table-top position with your calves parallel to the mat.

3. From this position, engage your abdominals and extend the opposite arm and leg away from each other, keeping them straight but diagonal to the mat and come back to the starting position.

4. Alternate with the other arm and leg. Repeat for 45 seconds.

**While extending your arm and leg, try not to move the opposite limbs.**

OR

**3A. MODIFICATION: MODIFIED HUNDRED PREP**

1. Lie supine on the mat with your hands straight up towards the ceiling, but in line with your shoulders. Bend your legs at the knees, feet on the floor.

2. From this position, inhale to prepare. On an exhale, lift your head, chest and shoulders off the mat, lower your arms towards your hips until they are hovering off the mat, reaching your fingertips away from you, and look between your legs.

3. Inhale and lower your head, chest and shoulders back towards the mat, with your hands towards the ceiling again.

4. Repeat Steps 2 and 3 for 45 seconds.

Break: 15 seconds.

**4. TEASER**

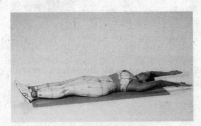 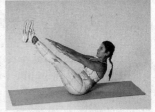

1.  Lie supine on your back with your arms and legs stretched straight out. Engage your abdominals so that you don't hyperextend your back.
2.  Inhale, lifting your head, circle your arms towards your feet and simultaneously lift your legs off the mat to form a gentle curve with your body, like a canoe.
3.  Exhale and float your body up to come into a Teaser.
4.  Take a full breath—inhale and exhale—while lowering your body back to the starting position with control.
5.  Repeat Steps 2 to 4 for 45 seconds.

OR

## 4A. MODIFICATION: MODIFIED TEASER

1.  Lie supine with your arms straight over your head.
2.  Lift your feet off the mat with your knees at a ninety-degree angle to reach the table-top position with your calves parallel to the mat.
3.  Inhale and exhale, circle your arms towards your feet, lifting your back off the mat while extending your legs at the same time to come up in a V-sit position. Keep your arms outstretched with your hands by your knees and your gaze straight.
4.  Roll back down to the mat bringing the legs to the table-top position.
5.  Repeat Steps 3 and 4 for 45 seconds.

**Make this even simpler without lifting your lower back, and just extending your legs and circling your arms to get them parallel to the mat.**

Break: 15 seconds.

## 5.   MOUNTAIN CLIMBERS

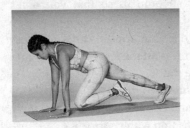 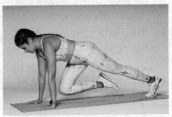

1.  Get into plank position by making sure that your wrists are under your shoulders, your body is in a straight line from your head to your heels, your abdominals are engaged and your glutes are squeezed.
2.  Keeping your upper body stable, bring one knee to the chest, and take it back.
3.  Bring the other knee to your chest and take it back.
4.  Alternate between legs and do the exercise at a good pace for 45 seconds for a good workout.

OR
## 5A. MODIFICATION: MOUNTAIN CLIMBER TAP

1.  Get into the plank position as in Step 1 above.
2.  From this position, without moving your upper body, bring your leg forward and tap your toes to the mat, and go back.
3.  Alternate with the other leg.
4.  Alternate between legs at a good pace for 45 seconds.

Break: 15 seconds.

*Repeat all five exercises to complete your 10-minute stack.*
*Full Body Stack 4 is done.*

## FULL BODY STACK 5

Full Body Stack 5 has five exercises. Each exercise will be done for 45 seconds with a 15-second break. Repeat once more to complete the 10-minute stack. You can either follow the steps below or use your phone to scan the QR code, and select  Full Body Stack 5 from the menu to work out along with me. Wherever possible, an easier, modified version of the exercises is also available.

### 1. SQUAT AND KICK

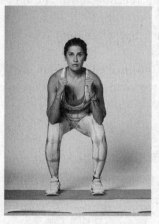 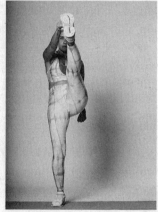

1. Stand upright with your feet shoulder-width apart and toes slightly turned out. Your fists must be in front of your chest and elbows down.
2. Flex at the hips, bend your knees to go down into a squat, keeping your chest open.
3. Extend your knees to come up and kick one leg in front of you, punching with the opposite hand.

4. Repeat the squat and kick with the other leg, punching with the opposite hand.
5. In this way, squat and kick, alternating legs for 45 seconds.

**You need not keep your fists in front of your chest as mentioned in Step 1, if it's too challenging. You can place your hands on your waist if you don't want to punch.**

OR

## 1A. MODIFICATION: SQUAT AND KNEE UP

1. Follow Steps 1 and 2 above.
2. From the squat, come up and bring your knee up, touching your knee with the opposite hand. Repeat the squat, come up and bring the other knee up, touching it with the opposite hand.
3. In this way, squat and knee up, alternating legs for 45 seconds.
4. You need not keep your fists in front of your chest as mentioned in Step 1, if it's too challenging. You can place your hands on your waist.

Break: 15 seconds.

## 2. ALTERNATE FORWARD RAISES IN PLANK

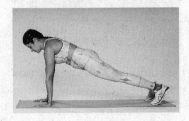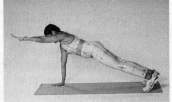

1. Get into the plank position. Make sure that your wrists are under your shoulders, your body is in a straight line from your head to your heels, your abdominals are engaged and your glutes are squeezed. Reach your heels away from you.

2.  From this position, lift one hand off, reaching it straight ahead in line with your shoulders and bring it back down on the mat. Repeat with the other hand.
3.  Keep alternating hands for 45 seconds.

**Try not to shift your weight too much.**

OR
## 2A. MODIFICATION: ALL-FOURS FORWARD REACHES

1.  Come into the all-fours position with wrists in line with your shoulders and knees in line with your hips. Keeping your back neutral, press into your hands to lift your shoulders away from the mat.
2.  From this position, lift one hand off, reaching it straight ahead in line with your shoulders and bring it back down on the mat. Repeat with the other hand.
3.  Keep alternating hands for 45 seconds.

Break: 15 seconds.

## 3.  BICYCLE

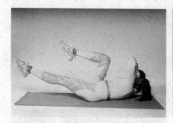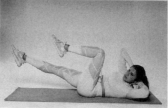

1.  Lie supine on the mat.
2.  Interlace your fingers and place them behind your head, keeping your elbows wide.

3.. Lift your feet off the mat, and bend your legs at the knees at a ninety-degree angle, with your calves parallel to the floor to reach the table-top position. Lift your head, chest and shoulders, and rest your head in your hands.

4. From this position, bend one knee while extending the other knee, simultaneously rotating your upper body towards your bent knee. And switch.

5. Alternate sides for 45 seconds.

**Keep your head lifted throughout the movement with your elbows wide.**

OR
**3A. MODIFICATION: ALTERNATE ELBOW TO KNEE**

1. Follow Steps 1 and 2 above.

2. Lift your feet off the mat, and bend your legs at the knees at a ninety-degree angle, with your calves parallel to the floor to reach the table-top position.

3. From this position, rotate your upper body towards the opposite knee and come back down.

4. Alternate for 45 seconds.

Break: 15 seconds.

**4. FROG BRIDGE PULSES**

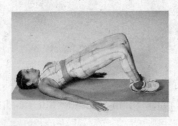 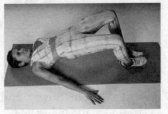

1. Lie supine on the mat, with your knees bent and feet together.
2. Keep your hands by your side on the mat in a V.
3. Pressing your heels together, take your knees away from each other.
4. Looking straight up, lift your hips up towards the ceiling.
5. Keeping your chest wide, squeeze and pulse your glutes up towards the ceiling, engaging your abdominals.
6. Pulse for 45 seconds and then bring your hips back down.

OR
## 4A. MODIFICATION: FROG BRIDGE

1. Follow Steps 1 to 3 above.
2. Looking straight up, lift your hips up towards the ceiling. And lower back down with control.
3. Repeat Step 2 for 45 seconds.

Break: 15 seconds.

## 5. PRONE LAT PULLS

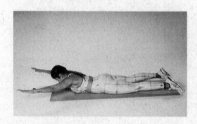 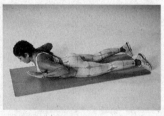

1. Lie prone on the mat with your arms and legs away from each other, abdominals engaged and glutes squeezed.
2. Sliding your shoulders away from your ears, lift your upper body off the mat.

3.  Bending your elbows towards your waist, imagine that you
    are pulling a rope behind your head.
4.  Extend your arms back out again to 'release' the rope, and
    pull back in again.
5.  Repeat for 45 seconds, keeping your upper body lifted and
    stable, and your abdominals engaged so that you relax your
    lower back.

Break: 15 seconds.

*Repeat all five exercises to complete your 10-minute stack.*
*Full Body Stack 5 is done.*

# Working It Out

## *Next Level*

### *That one habit that will take your workout to the next level*

What do you *want* from your workout? Toned arms, endurance, balance, flexibility, core strength, the ability to hold a plank for a minute? If you really want to achieve these, I'd like you to master a small, easy habit that could take your workout—and your results—to the next level.

*Start the exercise by visualizing the 'result' for that exercise.* Every time you do a push-up, think about your triceps and how you want them to look. With each crunch you perform, picture your abdominals looking toned and beach-ready (or however ready you want them to be). With every squat, picture how toned your thighs or glutes will look in those jeans. I guarantee you that this technique of visualization will change your workout dynamic and the energy with which you approach it. And that energy will fuel the intensity of your workout and get you quicker to where you want to be.

In Pilates, every session begins with the goal that we want to work towards—we visualize the body part, the exercises, the outcome. We go beyond the body and focus on aspects like breath, balance and engaging the core. Bringing the element of mindfulness to your workout will help you concentrate and see the result in your mind's eye. Your body will soon catch up.

# BONUS WORKOUTS

## Posture Stacks

For those of you who desire to have the ideal posture, it may be encouraging to know that very few of us actually have it. Most of us have some interpretation of it, none of which is ideal. The ideal posture is when your ear, shoulder, hip bone, knee and ankle are all in a straight, plumb line. Sometimes we even stand with one hip out, which loads one side of the body, causing imbalances.

Habits such as spending too much time looking at our phones or sitting at our desks can lead us to further deviate from the plumb line. Simply put, bad posture becomes our new posture. Designed in collaboration with ace physiotherapist Dr Hemakshi Basu, this bonus section is dedicated to all of us who are guilty of muscle imbalances and other postural transgressions, sometimes without even realizing it.

You can either follow the instructions listed in each exercise or scan the QR code and select the relevant Posture Stack from the menu to work out along with me.

# Fix Your Muscle Imbalance

Our muscles are designed in the form of sling systems which work diagonally across our body. Everything moves in synchronization—for example, our hips move in line with our shoulders. An imbalance in one part causes an imbalance in the other. An example of this would be when we talk with our phone to our ear and swing the other hand, which can cause a muscle imbalance between our anterior oblique chain and our posterior oblique chain. Our anterior oblique chain consists of the anterior muscles with opposite adductors and the posterior oblique chain consists of the latissimus dorsi and the glutes, which help rotate the muscles and swing the arms while walking. I would recommend that the following exercises be done by anyone who uses mobile phones, which means pretty much all of us.

You can either follow the instructions listed in each exercise below or scan the QR code, and select the Fix Your Muscle Imbalance stack from the menu to work out along with me.

## 1. OPPOSITE HAND TO KNEE PRESS

*To work the anterior oblique chain.*

1. Lie supine on the mat with your legs bent at the knees. From this position, lift one leg up to the table-top position (calf parallel to the mat) and place the opposite hand on the inside of the knee.
2. Lower your sternum to the floor and, engaging the adductors, exert equal and opposite pressure of the hand against the knee.
3. Hold for five counts, and relax. Switch sides and repeat.
4. Visually it may look like you're simply touching the knee, but your muscles are being engaged in opposition.

## 2. OPPOSITE HAND TO KNEE PRESS IN LOW BRIDGE

*To work the anterior and posterior oblique chains together.*

1. Lie supine on the mat with your legs bent at the knees. Lift your hips up just a few inches off the mat.
2. Keeping the hips lifted, lift one leg to the table-top position (calf parallel to the mat) and place the opposite hand against the knee. Exert equal and opposite pressure of the hand against the knee. Reach the arm and leg away from each other, keeping the knee bent. Push your knee gently for three seconds. Repeat five times.
3. Switch sides and repeat.

### 3. PRONE OPPOSITE HAND AND LEG RAISE

*To work the posterior oblique chain.*

1. Lie prone on the mat, with your arms and legs stretched out and away from each other. Make sure that your feet are hip-distance apart.
2. Lift and reach your opposite arm and leg away from each other, lifting your head so that your ear is parallel to your arm. Hold for 2–5 seconds and then lower down.
3. Alternate with the other leg and hand.
4. Repeat five times on each side.

Note: If you find lifting the opposite hands and legs challenging, then you can start by alternately lifting the arms, followed by alternately lifting the legs. Lastly, if you find yourself arching your back during the exercise, place a cushion under your pelvis, relax your back and continue the exercise.

## Fix Your Text Neck

I can say with confidence that there is no one reading this who is *not* guilty of spending too much time looking down at their phones, me included. Staring down at your phone or other devices can not only increase the weight of your head from an average of twelve kilos to an average of forty-eight kilos (the weight of an older school-going child) but can also load the joints and ligaments, lengthen and weaken the muscles, and load the discs of your cervical spine.

Here's a quick test to check if your neck is aligned or not. Stand upright and ask someone to take a picture of you from a side angle. If your ear is directly above your shoulder, give yourself a pat on the back. If your ear is ahead of your shoulder, do the following exercises that will better the alignment of your head, thereby correcting the condition known as Forward Head Syndrome, or 'text neck'.

You can either follow the instructions listed in each exercise below or scan the QR code, and select the Fix Your Text Neck stack from the menu to work out along with me.

## 1. CHIN GLIDES

*A mobility exercise to make sure the ears go over the shoulders.*

1. Put two fingers on your chin with gentle pressure. Glide your chin back, such that your ears go over your shoulders. Keep looking straight ahead, and hold for five counts. Glide back.
2. Repeat about six to ten times.
3. Take care to look straight ahead or focus your eyes on the horizontal plane—remember not to tilt your head up as it jams the joint nor tilt the chin down as it locks the neck.

## 2. ACTIVE CHIN GLIDES

1. Put two fingers on your chin. Glide your chin away from your fingers, hold for 5–10 counts and relax.
2. Repeat about six to ten times.
3. Take care as mentioned in (3) of the previous exercise.

## 3. STERNAL LIFT WITH HEAD ROTATION

1. Start in the all-fours position with your knees directly under your hips and wrists directly under your shoulders. Lift your chest away from the floor and get your head in line with the upper back.

2. Holding this position, rotate your head to the right and then to the left and relax.
3. Repeat six to ten times.

**The movements should be small: imagine you have a long pencil attached to your nose and you are making a line from left to right with your nose.**

## Fix Rounded Shoulders

DON'T SLOUCH! How often have you heard that? Slouching could lead to rounded shoulders, a rounded thoracic spine (mid-back), a rounded lumbar (lower back) spine and your head may feel like it is falling off your body.

Slouching leads to a plethora of chain reactions which include rounded shoulders, a rounded and therefore stiff thoracic spine, stiff shoulder and pectoralis muscles in the front, a shortened rectus abdominus and lengthened upper and lower back muscles making them less efficient, none of which are good for your body in the long term.

You can either follow the instructions listed in each exercise below or scan the QR code, and select the Fix Rounded Shoulders stack from the menu to work out along with me.

### 1. THORACIC ROTATION FOR UPPER BACK MOBILITY

1. Sit upright on a chair with your feet hip-width apart.
2. Put your hands together in a 'namaste' under your chin, keeping your fingers in line with your chin and nose.
3. Keeping your right hip grounded, rotate your torso as one unit to the left and come back to the centre and repeat on the other side.
4. Rotate six times on each side, coming back to the centre.

**Do remember not to move your neck beyond your fingers as that may injure your neck.**

## 2.    THORACIC ROTATION 2

1.  Sit upright on a chair with your feet hip-width apart and hands clasped behind your head. Hold the weight of your head in your hands and keep the elbows open.
2.  Twist from your waist and rotate to the right, feeling the stretch in your upper back. Come back to the centre and rotate to the left.
3.  Rotate six times on each side, coming back to the centre each time.

**Remember to keep the opposite hip grounded, and don't shrug your shoulders.**

## 3.    THE DART

1.  Lie prone on the mat and place a rolled napkin under your forehead. Keep your palms facing down on the mat to work in external rotation of the shoulder.
2.  Now, imagine holding a plum between your neck and your chin. Without squashing the imaginary plum, raise your shoulders slightly off the mat without retracting and lift both your arms off the floor for 5 to 10 seconds and lower back down.
3.  Repeat Step 2 for a total of six times.

**Keep the shoulders relaxed and arms close to your body.**

## 4.    REVERSE WALL V SLIDES

*Not recommended for people with shoulder injuries.*

1.  Stand with your back against a solid wall with your feet hip-width apart. Take a step forward and soften your knees

a little. Your back, head and shoulders should be relaxed. Draw your ribs towards the belly button and keep your head flat against the wall.

2. Start with your arms up against the wall in a W such that each elbow is in a V and your shoulders are externally rotated.

3. Keeping your ribs towards your belly button, slide your arms up the wall, keeping your wrist, forearm, elbow and arm connected to the wall at all times. Don't shrug your shoulders, and engage your core.

4. Lower the arms back to the starting position, maintaining the connection of the arms to the wall.

5. Repeat Steps 3 and 4 six times.

## 5.  SUPINE V SLIDES

*An easier version of the above exercise.*

1. Lie supine on the mat with your legs bent at the knees. Place a folded towel under your neck. Now, place your hands in the W position, palms facing up to externally rotate the shoulders.

2. From this position, slide your arms up the floor, keeping your wrist, forearm, elbow and arm connected to the floor. Don't shrug your shoulders. Engage your core, and go up only as much as you can without losing the connection of your arms to the floor.

3. Slide your arms down to the starting position.

4. Repeat Steps 2 and 3 six times, remembering to keep your chest and ribs down.

## Fix Your Lordotic Posture

Standing with your butt and belly sticking out? This means that your posture is lordotic—causing your hip flexors and back muscles to shorten, as well as your glutes and abdominals to lengthen and become inefficient, leading to backaches and loading the spine.

To fix a lordotic posture, lower your sternum towards your belly, squeeze your glutes to make sure that the pubis, belly and sternum are in one line. Remember not to slouch. That said, correcting a lordotic posture needs strengthening of the muscles, and the following three exercises are solutions to this very common problem.

You can either follow the instructions listed in each exercise below or scan the QR code, and select the Fix Your Lordotic Posture stack from the menu to work out along with me.

## 1. ARTICULATED GLUTE BRIDGE

1. Lie supine on the mat with your legs bent at the knees. Place a pillow between your knees, and squeeze it. Cross your hands over your chest and drop your sternum towards the floor.
2. From this position, squeeze your glutes to lift your hips up towards the ceiling in a low bridge, making sure that you do not lift your sternum off the mat, otherwise your back will arch and hurt. Squeezing the pillow, hold for a few counts and lower down.
3. Repeat Step 2 six times, making sure to keep the sternum and glutes engaged.

## 2. ALTERNATE LEG LIFTS

1. Lie supine on the mat with your legs bent at the knees and your arms by your side. Drop your ribs down towards the floor keeping your back flat on the mat.
2. From this position, lift one knee to ninety degrees, and place your foot back down.

3.  Alternate with the other leg.
4.  Repeat Steps 2 and 3 six times on each side, making sure that
    your back is flat on the floor, and that your pelvis is stable.

## 3.  PELVIC TILTS AGAINST THE WALL

*Having a lordotic posture means you have an anterior pelvic tilt,
which creates a big gap between the spine and the wall. To correct
this, do a posterior pelvic tilt against the wall.*

1.  Lean against a solid wall. Drop your sternum, engage the
    abdominals and the glutes to go into a posterior tilt. In other
    words, keep your spine flat and stuck against the wall.
2.  Hold for 3–5 counts and relax. Repeat six times.
3.  If you find this challenging, take a step forward and soften
    your knees.

## Wrist Strengthening

Are you in a high-wrist job? Strengthen
either or both wrists weakened by repetitive
movement. You can either follow the
instructions listed in each exercise below
or scan the QR code, and select the Wrist
Strengthening stack from the menu to work
out along with me.

## 1.  ALPHABET WITH THE WRIST

1.  Keeping the elbow stable, (support it with the other hand if
    you need to) and imagine you are holding a pen.
2.  Move the wrist to write alphabets in the air, all twenty-six of
    them (or those of a language of your choice).

## 2.  WRIST FLEXION STRETCH

1.  Put your thumb in your fist.
2.  Extend your hand in front of you at shoulder level and, with the other hand, gently pull your fist down feeling the stretch in the wrist. Hold for 3 seconds, and release.
3.  Repeat Step 2 five to ten times.

## 3.  WRIST EXTENSION STRETCH

1.  Stand with your side to a wall, at arms-length. Now, place the palm of your hand on the wall, with the fingers facing down. Your elbow should be straight.
2.  Relax your shoulders, and turn your body slightly away from the wall to feel the stretch in your wrist. Hold for 3 seconds, and release.
3.  Repeat Step 2 five to ten times.

# Desk Stretches

When you sit for long periods, it affects your body. No matter how conscious you are about sitting correctly, your spine will invariably not be where it is supposed to be, affecting your neck, back and body to a considerable degree. It is why it is often said that sitting is the new smoking.

These desk stretches can be done at, you guessed it, your desk. These are small, relatively unobtrusive movements that shouldn't alarm people around you.

You can either follow the instructions listed in each exercise below or scan the QR code, and select the Desk Stretches stack from the menu to work out along with me.

### 1.   NECK GLIDES

1.  Place two fingers on your chin and look diagonally down.
2.  Gently putting pressure on your chin, glide the neck back.
3.  Hold for 3–5 seconds and relax.
4.  Repeat five to ten times every few hours.

### 2.   SHOULDER AND CHEST STRETCH

1.  Sitting upright on a chair, interlace your fingers and place them behind your head, and move your elbows behind. This will enable your shoulders and chest to stretch.
2.  Hold for 3–5 seconds and relax.
3.  Repeat five to ten times every few hours.

### 3.   ARMS OPENER FOR THORACIC STRETCH

1.  Standing with your side to a wall, extend both your hands in front of you at shoulder level with the palms touching each other. Your arm should lightly brush against the wall.
2.  Keeping the hand close to the wall and the pelvis stable, rotate the torso reaching your other arm away from you maintaining it at shoulder level.
3.  Bring it back to the starting position.
4.  Repeat three to five times and change sides.

### 4.   FULL SPINE STRETCH

1.  Facing a table, hinge at the hips to place your hands on the table.
2.  Keeping your knees soft, reach your tailbone and fingertips away from each other to feel the stretch in your back and repeat.
3.  Repeat Step 2 three to five times every few hours.

## 5.  ANKLE CIRCLES

1. Sitting upright on a chair with your knees bent, reach one leg straight out in front of you hovering off the floor.
2. Circle the foot in a clockwise and then an anti-clockwise direction.
3. Repeat five to ten times for each ankle every few hours.

## FITNESS STORIES

**Sophie Choudry**

*I am Flaw-some*

Growing up in London, I never really had body issues; I was a size 8–10, and that was fine. But when I came to India to video jockey (VJ) at MTV and act in films, I began to have an awareness of my body that I never had before. Whether it was being surrounded by women with skinnier frames or stylists trying to cover up my 'flaws', I began to feel more self-conscious and insecure about how I looked. That was then. I am now the most confident I have ever been. Reaching this point has partly to do with my fitness but also with learning to enjoy my perfections and imperfections because we all have them.

I started working out with Yasmin about ten years ago when I had a neck slipped disc and other related issues and needed help with rehabilitation. We got connected through a friend, and I decided to try one class. Of course, by the end of it, I realized very quickly that Yasmin knew what she was talking about. With the help of my physiotherapist Dr Hemakshi Basu and Yasmin, I not only became fit enough within a few months to shoot a hit song opposite John Abraham in *Shootout at Wadala* but also later take part, and thrive, in *Jhalak Dikhlaja*, which was more like a stunt show than a dance show! Nobody could tell that I had gone through so much to do it.

Fitness is a journey, but it isn't always a smooth one—travelling, events, eating out, celebrations can tinker with the delicate balance you need to achieve to maintain both your weight and your fitness levels. Motivation can also play hide-and-seek. While I was the fittest I have ever been during the first lockdown thanks to Yasmin's online sessions, the second lockdown was an entirely different story. I was so consumed by the devastation around me that working out was the last thing on my mind. It is only when things got better that I got back to the gym.

If I could put my fitness philosophy in one word, it is consistency—showing up for myself almost every day. And that consistency is founded on finding workouts I love, and eating healthfully but not restrictively. Working out regularly also keeps me mentally sane and happy. If you want to see long-term results, you must make fitness a part of your life. I am fitter now than I was in my twenties, and I have a lot of body confidence. I would like to say that I am 'flaw-some'—I have flaws but I still feel amazing because I'm 'me', and I think it's really important for all of us to grow to that stage. The last two years have taught us that there is nothing more important than our health. Fitness is all about how you feel inside.

## Saman Ali Khan

*Fitness can change the way you deal with life.*

When my husband Irfan was diagnosed with Stage IV lung cancer, it changed our lives forever. As a decision-maker and caregiver, and also a wife, mother and partner at work, I came under tremendous pressure, both mental and physical. I was unsettled, restless, irritable, exhausted and just by chance, came upon these wonderful lines: 'When you can't control what's happening, challenge yourself to control the way you respond to what's happening. That's where your power is."

I needed to do just that, and the way to do it was be fit, both mentally and physically. I have always been a sportswoman, so the gym felt like a homecoming in a way. The challenge, though, was to start afresh at the age of sixty. And thus began my journey with Yasmin at YKBI in 2017.

Meeting Yasmin opened up a completely new vista. She understood my mental state along with my physical form and patiently gave me an insight into her vision of fitness. She, along with my gym instructor Akash and the entire team at the studio, continuously and untiringly encouraged me, through all the ups and downs in my personal life as well. It is inconceivable to think that in a short span of a month or two, I could feel the change both internally and externally, but I did—it was like the layers of anxiety, stress, fear, aches and pains were peeling off. My body language transformed—the gait, the posture, the confidence.

'For a seed to achieve its greatest expression, it must come completely undone.'† Only then it can grow. For me it was the same—I completely surrendered and then emerged empowered. I lost Irfan in 2021, but this new me could cope and carry on despite the huge loss, which is why for me fitness is a way to face life, with all its joys and sorrows.

---

* 'When you can't control what's happening, challenge yourself to control the way you respond to what's happening. That's where your power is,' *Improve My World*, accessed 11 December 2022, https://www.improvemyworld.com/when-you-cant-control-whats-happening-challenge-yourself-to-control-the-way-you-respond-to-whats-happening-thats-where-your-power-is/

† 'For a seed to achieve its greatest expression, it must come completely undone. The shell cracks, its insides come out and everything changes. To someone who doesn't understand growth, it would look like complete destruction,' Pass It On, accessed 11 December 2022, https://www.passiton.com/inspirational-quotes/7876-for-a-seed-to-achieve-its-greatest-expression

# PART THREE: FITNESS TIPS AND TRICKS

# 4

# Fitness Plateaus

## *The glass ceilings of fitness and how to SMASH\*N your way through*

There comes a time in almost everyone's fitness journey when our results flatline—a line so straight we could do chin-ups on it. And no matter what we do to get fitter or leaner, it doesn't seem to work. The weight stays the same, the fitness levels stay the same, we look the same and our progress 'plateaus'.

Bodies are intelligent, responsive things. Too much of the same, and they adapt. It's one of the reasons we gain even more weight after crash-dieting—the body thinks it's not getting enough food and it starts storing more of what we eat as fat, almost like insurance for future energy expenditure.

This line best explains plateaus with weight training, 'once your central nervous system has learnt to recruit all the muscle fibres it needs to complete a given number of reps, it stops adding new muscle because it can do the job you've asked of it with what it has.'[*] Similarly, we also expend less energy while doing the

---

[*] '5 Training Strategies That'll Make Sure You Never Plateau,' *Men's Journal*, accessed 12 October 2022, https://www.mensjournal.com/health-fitness/5-ways-to-long-term-fitness-success/.

same cardio workout* day after day, which leads us to the natural conclusion that fitness's secret weapon is *the element of surprise*. I like to call a plateau the *glass ceiling of fitness*, where your goal seems within reach, but something is preventing you from getting there. My foray into Pilates was precisely that—to bring in the element of surprise because no matter what I did after my second baby—crunches, cardio, weightlifting, crying—I couldn't shake off my belly fat. I knew that my body needed something new. I researched options, discovered the potential of Pilates, got my certification, broke my plateau and also started introducing it to my clients. It opened up a whole new world for me and for the clients I trained.

That said, when we feel we have hit a plateau, *it may not be a plateau at all*. The first thing I usually advise clients when they come to me with their woes is to have an honest conversation with the one person that has the biggest impact on their fitness—themselves.

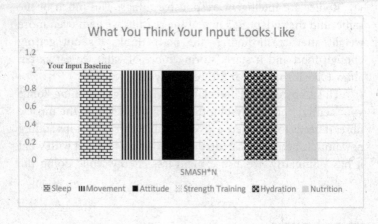

* 'Seven Ways to Break a Fitness Plateau,' *Lark*, accessed 12 October 2022, https://www.lark.com/blog/seven-ways-to-break-a-fitness-plateau/.

A plateau occurs when you *think* you are putting in the same input, and not getting any significant results or output. If I have learnt anything after thirty years in the business, it is that there is *rarely* a case where progress has stalled despite someone doing all that they can. In almost all cases, people have unconsciously stepped back from the healthy habits that got them to their goals.

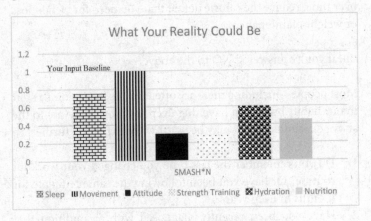

What Your Reality Could Be

If you feel your progress has stalled, ask yourself:

1. Has travel, a wedding or a stressful period at work disrupted your mealtimes?
2. Have you been working out with reduced intensity? Have more breaks between workouts crept in?
3. Have you been doing too much cardio, and not enough strength training?
4. Has disinterest crept into your workout? This could mean, for example, that you aren't motivated enough to increase your weights while doing resistance exercises.
5. Are you not sleeping as well as you used to?
6. Are you not drinking as much water as you used to?

If you've answered *yes* to any or all the above, then it's not a plateau but a subtle shift in your routine that may have gone unnoticed. Fitness and weight management can sometimes be about achieving a delicate balance, and even minor changes in your habits over the long term—extra calories consumed over the weekend or more missed workouts—can stagnate your progress. An extra spoonful of sugar in your tea or coffee can, over time, reduce the calorie deficit that you need for weight loss or weight maintenance.

But if you've answered NO to the above:

Most people—including me—are often unable to pinpoint a shift in our habits but if you have dug deep and answered 'no' to the above questions then it may be worthwhile exploring further:

1. Do you remember the last time you changed your workout routine? Or have you been following the same template for months or even years?
2. Have you been recently diagnosed with a condition that impacts your metabolism?
3. Are you over forty? To maintain the same fitness levels, you may need to do different things.
4. Are you working out *too* hard? Take more rest days. Over-exercising is not only dangerous but counterproductive.

Whether your self-assessment is accurate or not, it's always time for a change. And to get different results, you have to do things differently. But changes don't necessarily have to be radical. The example on the next page explains how you can break the stalemate without increasing your workout time.

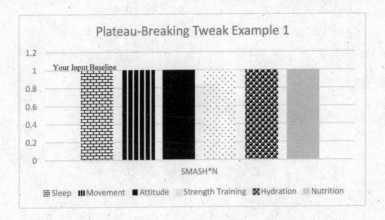

This tweak involves restoring your regular sleeping, hydration, strength training and nutritional habits. If you go for a walk regularly, increase the intensity (marked in thicker stripes) by taking more steps or give yourself a challenge by walking up and down hilly roads. Add some skipping or running to your routine, if possible. You could also replace a walking session with swimming or cycling.

Another way to break a plateau is to increase the amount of strength training whilst reducing the amount of cardio. Additionally, make healthy and sustainable nutritional changes by including more fibre, vegetables, fruit or protein, by changing your carbohydrates around or eating less junk. That said, if you have an underlying medical condition or might be allergic to certain foods, I recommend that any dietary changes be made under professional supervision. Here's one more example of a tweak:

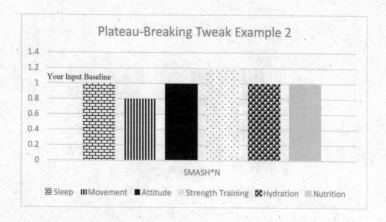

Conversely, you could also replace an hour or two of gym training with another kind of workout like circuit training, which is usually part cardio. Your body will need to use different muscles and work harder to do what you're telling it to do.

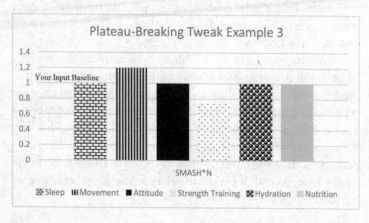

While I've given you three examples of tweaks, the combinations are, of course, endless. You can also increase your overall workout time or overhaul your diet significantly if smaller changes aren't working. Or stop everything and do something completely new. But do keep in mind that:

*You will only see progress by surprising your body.*

\*

## Bumps that Feel Like Plateaus

When is plateau not a plateau? While I am quite sure that this is not a question that keeps you up at night, there are times when your progress is halted by what *feels* like a plateau but are life events that lead you to miscalculate or lose momentum. I thought I'd list them in no particular order:

**Childbirth and breastfeeding:** Babies are joyful, yes, but getting them from Point A (inside your body) to Point B (outside your body) can turn the body inside out. Childbirth is both a magical and traumatic time and I know no woman who has pushed out a baby and uttered the words, 'Well, that was something, wasn't it? Now, who's going to drive me to the gym?'

Post-partum healing is a complicated, emotional and a highly individualistic process, and the last thing any mother should be thinking of is about fitness or 'getting her body back'. Her immediate priorities must be to take of herself and her baby. Barring a few cases, almost everyone I know has battled with post-partum weight gain, so I say to the mother reading this that she is not alone. She must also realize that it took her nine months to prepare for this moment, and it will take her at least nine months till she feels like herself again. To her I prescribe patience and understanding.

Now, of course, there is greater awareness about weight gain during pregnancy and doctors frown upon too much of it for fear of other complications. I had gained about twenty-five kilos during each of my pregnancies, so when I delivered my boys, I was still about twenty kilos overweight, both times. What helped me get back in shape was giving up processed sugar—there's no nutritional benefit in processed sugar—but still eating healthfully enough to breastfeed my babies. I'd make some healthy substitutions so when making sheera, I'd get it cooked with gud (instead of sugar), raisins and water (instead of milk). I'd similarly swap wheat for jowar, white rice for brown rice, and so on. But the one thing I wouldn't do is compromise on eating well, because I was the primary food source for a tiny human being, and for myself, of course.

That said, we cannot ignore the fact that breastfeeding makes you hungry . . . like climb-on-the-walls hungry, like my-husband-looks-like-a-walking-pizza hungry. Underestimating what you're eating is also common because most mothers are exhausted, sleep-deprived, and the last thing they're thinking of while rummaging around in the fridge at 2 a.m. is whether the cold roti they're chewing on is jowar, bajra or cardboard. Don't spend time worrying too much about weight gain in the immediate post-partum phase, and *never* start working out until you're cleared by your doctor to do so.

**Menopause:** Menopause is that time in a woman's life when she feels overwhelmed and not in control of her life. Sudden weight gain, maldistribution of fat, abdominal weight gain (because of oestrogen deficiency), mood swings, hot flashes, irritability, depression and other sometimes sudden and alarming symptoms are hardly conducive to putting on stretchy pants and cheerfully heading out for a run. Menopausal women also often have disturbed sleep, which leads to the excess release of cortisol, further adding to belly fat. Exercise, good nutrition and core strengthening are some of the best ways to manage this phase. That said, do start only when you are ready to and until then, be kind to yourself.

**Significant life events:** Traumatic or difficult life events like the loss of a job, death of a loved one, stress at work, divorce, an unexpected diagnosis are not what I would term ideal conditions for thinking about your next fitness move. Here is where I would recommend that you just keep things simple, like going for a walk if you're feeling up to it, or generally taking care of your mental well-being. This is your time to heal, and everyone heals differently.

**Post injury or surgical procedures:** When I had torn my anterior cruciate ligament (ACL)—during an incident that was entirely my fault—I was not allowed to work out for a *long* time. Imprisoned by the consequences of my own actions, I decided to do the next best thing—be as careful with food as possible. It didn't help that medication made me hungrier or the less I moved, the hungrier I felt. Preparing meals ahead of time really helped me during that phase because when we're sitting at home, thoughts tend to turn towards food especially if there's nothing much else to do. Arming myself with hummus and vegetables, nuts and fruits ahead of time, helped me with the cravings.

**Forced changes in routine:** Any significant change in routine could mess with a system that took time to perfect, which could have unintended consequences. For sportspeople, it's the off-season when athletes gain weight. For working professionals, it could be a period of travel. During the lockdown, people either gained weight or got fit.

While bumps have a way of sorting themselves out, breaking plateaus is a matter of trial and error and I recommend you keep the SMASH*N approach as a base to work from. Treat sleep and attitude as 'constant'—they should be as complete and as positive as can be—and play around with the other four 'variables'. And do give yourself a few weeks or months for changes to kick in.

If the surprises you're introducing to your body are surprising you by their lack of result, consult a professional. They'll give you more ideas after doing a thorough assessment of your body. Stay strong and be patient (the A of SMASH*N), and things will turn around. I say this with confidence because throughout my career, what I have seen is that no matter how stubborn my clients' plateau is, they always break out of it in the end.

## FITNESS STORIES

### Aaliyah Qureishi

*Fitness has to be sustainable.*

Yasmin Karachiwala, my *jiji*, my aunt, has not only been a fitness inspiration but has also changed the way I see fitness—making me realize that exercise is not a way of punishing my body but celebrating it. From coming in to YKBI when I was twelve and skinny—and still thinking I was fat—to being toned, fit, strong and confident, I feel I have come a long way.

But this has not been a journey without setbacks. When I left home to study, I didn't have access to the gym I was so familiar with. I was grappling with a new environment, a new system, the stress of exams, and had access mainly to junk food. I was gaining weight and I felt I had no control over my body.

Setbacks can feel like the end of the world, but my way of dealing with them was by taking it one workout at a time. My fitness philosophy is to do something I love because only then it will be sustainable, and to eat to nourish the body. My aunt always says that 70 per cent of the body is built in the kitchen and not in the gym, so eating clean is important to me. This doesn't mean that I don't get off my regime sometimes because it is equally important to listen to my body.

*

**Alizeh Agnihotri**

*Results come when you have the mindset.*

I have had the privilege of knowing Yasmin my whole life. She encouraged, but never pressured me, to work out until I had achieved the right mindset. Exercising is something that no one can force you to do, you need to make that decision on your own but once you're committed, nothing can stop you.

Initially, my goal was superficial—I worked out to lose weight. But once I actually got into a proper workout routine, I understood that fitness and well-being were so much more than just being skinny. It was about feeling your best and your strongest; inside and out. I always take the time out to go to the gym, no matter how busy or tired I am. It's my 'me' time, and I always feel better after exercising. I have realized that maintenance is much more important and long-lasting than achieving temporary goals.

My journey has been far from perfect, but it's important to accept that, like Rome, your body isn't built in a day. It is frustrating and tiring, but being on a fitness track doesn't mean that you have to stop enjoying your life; you just have to create a plan that makes you happy. But do start. 'A journey of a thousand miles begins with a single step,'* and the journey to fitness begins with just 10 minutes.

*

* 'Lao Tzu,' *BBC*, accessed 8 December 2022, https://www.bbc.co.uk/worldservice/learningenglish/movingwords/shortlist/laotzu.shtml.

5

# The Big Bang Fitness Menu

## *Exploring the fitness explosion in the post-pandemic world*

The versatility of the 10-minute workout stacks outlined in *The Perfect 10: 10-Minute Workouts You Can Do Anywhere* lies in the fact that they can not only be stacked with each other but also with other fitness technologies and techniques. Did I hear you wanted a half-hour swim after a three-stack workout? Or squeeze in a Pilates class followed by a cool-down stack? You go for it, I say. Stack, bookend, squeeze, pad—the beauty of fitness is that it can be broken down or supersized to suit your unique needs.

While the pre-2020 world of fitness was already vast, the COVID-19 pandemic opened a whole new universe of online and home workouts, the Big Bang of Fitness, as it were. Vast has now upsized to limitless and new techniques, trends and classes are being added all the time. Online workouts have given people the flexibility they never had before. A client of mine wasn't making her in-person classes and held her travel schedule responsible. But her perfectly reasonable explanation of *I'm barely in town* no longer resonated in the post-pandemic era. All she had to do was flip open her laptop in Bahrain, Belize or Bengaluru, and there I'd be. *Squeeze your glutes, engage your abdominals.*

Online, in-person, in the pool, on the road, suspended from the ceiling, jumping on a trampoline, you can now work out anywhere and anyhow at your convenience, which sounds incredible, outrageous even; a whole new world of workouts, bursting with possibility, hope, depth and dimension.

It also sounds exhausting. If you feel that you are drowning in choice, treat this as a bit of a life raft. *The Big Bang Fitness Menu* has been culled from what's available and trending in the post-pandemic fitness universe in India and globally so that you can make an informed decision. You may see some old friends on this list,* it is in no particular order and neither is it exhaustive, but it includes updated trends and workout tips. You can stack these either with the 10-minute stacks in this book or dip into these by themselves on some days, or both. The post-pandemic world is your oyster.

That said, wherever you are on the fitness spectrum, you need to remember that your fitness approach must consist of *six* key elements, and the first four are concerned with the workout itself. These are:

-W- **Strength**

~ **Flexibility**

🕑 **Endurance**

🔋 **Rest**

*Strength* is resistance training and weightlifting, which will help you build muscle and burn calories at rest. This can be achieved using your own body weight, free weights, gym weight machines, machines like the Pilates reformer, and others. Depending upon

---

* 'Worldwide Survey of Fitness Trends for 2022,' *ACSM's Health and Fitness Journal*, accessed 12 October 2022, https://journals.lww.com/acsm-healthfitness/Fulltext/2022/01000/Worldwide_Survey_of_Fitness_Trends_for_2022.6.aspx.

your goals—strength, toning, muscle definition—you can have more or less of this in your workout week, but it can't be done away with entirely.

I also must add here that a healthy muscle is a *supple* muscle, not one that is in constant contraction. Contrary to popular opinion, when you see these super-built-up ~~houses~~ humans walking around with their muscles popping out, it is *not* healthy. A healthy muscle should be supple to touch, but when flexed, should be hard as a rock, which brings me to my next point.

*Flexibility* is defined as 'the ability of a joint or series of joints to move through an unrestricted, pain-free range of motion.'*And it is that very flexible range of motion that protects you from injuring your joints or your back during routine everyday tasks or recovering faster when you do. When your muscles are hard and tight, they can develop tears—stretching them or doing workouts like Pilates or yoga help build flexibility.

*Endurance* is cardiovascular exercise which will raise your heartbeat and build stamina. It is also great for fat burning and weight loss, although in a different way from resistance training. Again, how much of it you do in a week depends on your goals, but endurance is not something that you can completely do without either.

*Rest* is a break from working out, but the importance of this is often underestimated or is at odds with a fitness culture that often equates gain with pain. I am here to tell you that there is *nothing* to be gained from pain. Rest is crucial both for your body to show improvements, and to recover in time for your next workout. This, of course, doesn't mean that you work out for one day a week and rest for six, but you know where I'm going with this.

---

* 'Flexibility,' *Physiopedia*, accessed 12 October 2022, https://www. physio-pedia.com/Flexibility#:~:text=Flexibility%20is%20the%20 ability%20of,joint%20and%20total%20body%20health.

Fifth, you also need **Quality**.

*Quality* refers to working with certified trainers or instructors and choosing appropriate workout gear to give you comfort. It also means maintaining the correct workout form to avoid injury—it's always better to do fewer reps with the correct form than doing many reps with incorrect form.

And lastly, you need **Consistency**. ⊙

Getting into shape, getting off medication or hitting fitness goals like doing push-ups, hikes or planking can be achieved if you commit to a time and place to do them. And do them often.

Where needed, I'll be using these six icons ⊸⋀⋁⋏⊷ ⊙ ✿ 💤 ∼ 💧 throughout the chapter to indicate the relative benefits of that workout or equipment, as well as tips on maintaining quality and consistency.

## 1. Group exercise classes—online and offline

Group exercise was how I started my career—doing a Jane Fonda-style of VHS aerobics that was popular back then. In post-pandemic India, you can continue to opt for spinning, Pilates, body conditioning, Bollywood dance, Zumba and even something called barre (pronounced 'bar'), although I suspect no drinking will be permitted.

Best suited for those who don't like working out alone, group classes are enjoyable, motivating, bring about a sense of community and are gently competitive, helping you stay on track. There are also equipment-led group Pilates classes, which makes Pilates more affordable.

While some of these may seem familiar, the difference is that many class options are now available online, with a range of timings to suit the early-riser and the late-sleeper. If you are looking at online options, do remember that you can access group classes from all over the world, so depending on budget and time zone, you can introduce more variety into your regime. And of course, fun, which is the main point.

~ ⏱ ⎼ᴧᴧ⎯ Group classes can be good for strength, flexibility or endurance training, so make sure to discuss your goals with your trainer.

🏅 Please do your quality checks by looking at ratings, reviews, certifications of the instructors like the American Council of Exercise (ACE) Group Instructor Certification, or other similar group instructor certifications, and of course, relying on your instinct when you walk into a studio for in-person classes. If the place is looking shabby or the equipment is not lovingly maintained or you just don't get a good 'vibe', look elsewhere.

◎ To maintain consistency, try to do a group class at a fixed time each time, either online or offline. You can also get a workout buddy to keep you accountable. Like gym memberships, offline classes should be either close to your house or place of work. If it's too far or inconvenient to get to, you are not going to go.

## 2. HIIT and Tabata

Already popular pre-pandemic and one of my favourite kinds of training, HIIT (High Intensity Interval Training) involves performing a particular exercise—any exercise—for 40–45 seconds with a 15–20 second break, to complete a minute. Tabata is a kind of HIIT but it has a more compact exercise: break ratio with 20 seconds of exercise and a 10-second break.

Both HIIT and Tabata's high-intensity-short-break formats help you burn more calories with the same exercise and have numerous other health benefits, which is why the workouts prescribed in the 10-minute stacks also use the HIIT format. HIIT can be done within group classes, gyms or personal training and has been designed to maximize the effects of the exercise you perform.

~ 🕐 –⋀⋁⋀– This is also suitable for all three, depending on whether the exercises are strength, flexibility or endurance-oriented.

◎🎖 To maintain consistency and quality, try the tips mentioned on page 271.

## 3. Home Gyms

Great for people who are short on time or who prefer to work out alone, home gyms have also gained in popularity post-pandemic. However, I do recommend that you get a qualified instructor to check your form. In my experience, those who can afford a home gym can usually afford an instructor, and supervised instruction is always better than no instruction. If you don't want the instructor to come home, you can request for an online class.

~ 🕐 –⋀⋁⋀– Depending on the budget, home gyms may not have endurance equipment like treadmills, elliptical machines and so on, but you can always invest in a skipping rope, an aerobic stepper or other low-cost but effective cardio solutions.

How you want to structure your home gym experience depends upon your goals.

I always advise people to invest in quality equipment from reputed companies and a good trainer with either American Council of Exercise (ACE), or National Academy of Sports Medicine (NASM), or National Strength and Conditioning Association (NSCA), or K11 (India) or American College of Sports Medicine (ACSM) certification. Beware of any customs duties for equipment though, which contribute to delivery delays and hidden costs.

To maintain consistency, set reasonable and measurable goals with your trainer or workout buddy that you can be held accountable for.

## 4.  Smart Bikes

The demand for smart stationary bikes exploded globally during the pandemic. Trapped in their homes and hooked up to online instructors leading a vibrant community, people were able to get a great cardio workout with many hitting their fitness and weight loss targets. Depending on how advanced your workout levels are, you can choose from airdyne, spinning or other bikes designed for professionals, as well as people with limitations. There are also recumbent bikes, which are safe for hip joints, knees and backs.

Smart bikes are great for cardio workouts with some strength benefits. Take care to adjust your seat to get the best form and prevent damage to your back, knees and hips.

Online reviews, conversations with gym instructors and going to sports stores will help you make an informed decision.

Beware of any customs duties if importing a bike, which could
add to hidden costs and delivery delays.

⊙ The group option to smart bikes is a spinning class and
there's nothing like flashing lights, pumping music and healthy
competition to give you something to look forward to and
keep you on track. If you prefer going at it alone, online bike
instructors may help you get the best out of your workout.

## 5.  Outdoor Activities and Sports

Outdoor activities are a great way to work out without *feeling*
like you're working out—and are some of the easiest, most
cost-effective ways to get fit. Swimming, cycling, running and
so on all have their own unique but tremendous benefits—but
make sure to mix these up as mentioned in *Fingers 1, Bodies
0,* and maybe combine a walk with a swim, for example, to see
results. Do note that you can only get calorie-burn benefits
from outdoor activities after 20 minutes of consistent exercise,
whether outdoors or indoors.

~ ⏱ -W- Outdoor activities include hiking, skipping,
swimming, cycling, kayaking, tennis, table tennis, sailing, squash,
golf, cricket, badminton, football, but this list is not exhaustive.
Depending on your goal—or just your passion—you can choose
activities that build strength, flexibility and endurance in
different ways, but my experience is that most people do these
for the sheer love of it.

🏅 The best way to have a good quality outdoor workout is
to be present and enjoy the feeling of being outdoors. For those
with a competitive streak, having a regular group to play sports
with—or against—is a good way to get the best out of it, if that's
what you so desire.

⊙ If you want to stick to an outdoor activity, start with something you like and see if it becomes something you eventually love. The bonus is finding your 'fitness tribe'—people who you can do these activities with, who love them as much as you do.

## 6. Wearable Technology

This includes pedometers, smart watches, fitness trackers and other wearable gadgets that track heart rate, steps taken, and other fitness parameters. To me, these have been a great way to track my movement outside of the classes I conduct and motivate me to go that extra mile. Consciousness is completion for me, and these gadgets help me squeeze in some movement where I otherwise would not have—on vacation, while running errands and walking short distances instead of driving.

In my experience, they also work very well when you follow the something-is-better-than-nothing philosophy. Small increments in steps added, add up to your overall calorie burn, and you might have a nice surprise waiting for you at your next weigh-in.

These are also great for senior citizens because as they get older, their lifestyles get more sedentary. My mother has one. Owing to her age, I've given her a target of 3000–5000 steps per day, which she completes by getting up every few hours and walking around the house.

Wearable technology is often associated with counting steps or monitoring heart rates, but now there's stuff for resistance training too. Some smart watches not only count the number of reps while weight training, but also have muscle heat maps to help you track the areas you're focusing on.

~ ⏱ –〰️– Wearable technology serves resistance, flexibility and endurance needs, but you can choose simpler options, depending upon your budget. If you only want the gadget to track your steps, you can choose a more cost-effective option, or even just use your phone with a step counting app (although it may not be as accurate). Many also come with their own apps.

🎖 Given the size of the community, you should be able to access many reviews about brands and do a cost-benefit comparison. It doesn't hurt to ask a few friends, too.

◎ By making you conscious of your workouts and your exercise history, these are deigned to build consistency. All you have to do is remember to put it on.

## 7. Fitness Apps

What strikes me about today's fitness apps is how inclusive they are and how quickly they've improved over a period of just a few years. There's something for everyone. If I were to construct a fitness app, I would not only have to put Pilates and other exercises on it, but also cater to audiences who like yoga, dancing, Zumba, weightlifting, walking, running, amongst other features. Some apps even have walking exercises that you can do *in place:* like marching, marching with knees up, moving from side-to-side, and so on. And all good apps come with nutritional tracking.

~ ⏱ –〰️– Fitness apps, like wearable technology, can also provide options for resistance, flexibility and endurance tracking.

Finding the right app for you is a process of trial and error, but the relative cost is low. Learn to weed out the unhelpful ones early.

Don't forget to turn on app notifications or customize the settings to suit your goals—it'll help you be more consistent.

## 8.  Strength Training with Free Weights

Free weights—like dumbbells, ankle weights, barbells, weighted balls, kettlebells—are a great in-between option for those who do not have the space or resources for a home gym but still want to scale up their workouts. Free weights give you the ability to do so many more functional movements over and above gym machines, which make them both convenient and versatile.

That said and I say again, form is extremely important, especially with weights. Always try to work with a certified instructor to get the form right before you branch off on your own and always, *always* start with lighter weights. Ask your trainer if you can take videos of them demonstrating the exercise. Too much too soon can and will injure you.

Depending on the workout, free weight training can also build flexibility as well as strength.

For a quality workout, choose a trainer with either American Council of Exercise (ACE), or National Academy of Sports Medicine (NASM), or National Strength and Conditioning Association (NSCA), or K11 (India) or American College of Sports Medicine (ACSM) certification.

◎ Gently increase the weight and the difficulty-level. If you feel your workout is too hard, it may discourage you from being more consistent.

## 9. Body Weight Training

A subset of strength training, body weight training is when you're using your own body weight against you—push-ups and pull-ups are good examples. You'd be surprised at how challenging it can be. For example, it may be harder to do a push-up than a chest press—you can always experiment with the weight you're pumping but you don't have a choice in the matter of your own body weight. The best part about it is that once you get your form sorted, you can do body weight training *anywhere*.

~ ⏱ –⋀⋁⋀– Body weight training is especially good for resistance and flexibility. Done in an HIIT or cardio format, it can also be good for building endurance.

🏅 Pick a trainer with either American Council of Exercise (ACE), or National Academy of Sports Medicine (NASM), or National Strength and Conditioning Association (NSCA), or K11 (India) or American College of Sports Medicine (ACSM) certification.

◎ Like free weight training, start slow. Start with the modified version of the exercise, and then work up to the intermediate and advanced levels. Too much too soon can discourage you from progressing further.

## 10. Personal Training

Always a good option for those who prefer working out alone or prefer one-on-one attention, a good personal trainer can get you into a shape you never thought you could achieve. Take your time and shop for the right trainer—you don't have to work with the first one you paired with. I always ask potential clients to try a couple before they commit to one. A good working relationship on the training floor will always give the best results.

What puzzles me is how reluctant people are to ask their trainer if they are certified. Certification is *very* important and the trainer must at least have ACE or ACSM certification, or it's not worth pursuing the conversation. Don't be shy or hesitate to ask them to show it to you because your body is literally in their hands.

~ ⏱ –〰– The world is your oyster when it comes to personal training. You can customize your workout to suit your goals or change course when it's not working.

🎖 Pick a trainer with either American Council of Exercise (ACE), or National Academy of Sports Medicine (NASM), or National Strength and Conditioning Association (NSCA), or K11 (India) or American College of Sports Medicine (ACSM) certification.

◉ Personal trainers are especially invested in your progress, and the good ones design workouts that you can enjoy.

## 11. Health and Wellness Coaching

Health and wellness coaching concerns itself with the relationship between your mental well-being, spiritual development and health goals. These coaches differ from trainers or nutritionists, in that they specialize in behavioural change—whether it's losing weight, getting fitter, quitting smoking or reducing your alcohol intake. Getting a good coach could help you achieve goals you never thought you could.

◎ While these don't directly train you, they will help you be more consistent.

🏅 Please do pick a coach with the ideal certification, but do also make sure you ask around, read the reviews and settle on someone only after you're confident it's the right fit.

## 12. Yoga

We all know that yoga has tremendous mind-body benefits, cementing its place in the post-pandemic Big Bang Fitness world as a global, leading fitness option. Depending on the school of yoga and the kind of class, it is great for endurance, flexibility and resistance training, and can again be safely practiced both online and in-person, alone or in a group. Elaborating on the myriad and wonderful benefits of yoga is the subject of a whole other book, and a short paragraph doesn't do it justice. But I'll just leave you with some popular schools that have worked for people: *kundalini*, *ashtanga*, *hatha*, *Iyengar*, to name just a few.

∼ ⏱ ⎯〜⎯ Depending on the asana and the intensity, it can be great for resistance, endurance and flexibility.

🏅 Don't be afraid to ask for the yoga teacher's qualifications. There are a great many yoga institutions in this country, and many have their own vigorous vetting process.

◎ As with everything else, consistency in your yoga practice is key to your progress. Luckily, you have access to a whole range of yoga formats from personal training to group classes to online training to retreats, all of which give you multiple options to choose from.

## 13. Pilates

Created by Joseph Pilates in the early part of the twentieth century, Pilates was so far ahead of its time that it didn't begin to achieve its now well-deserved recognition until the first few years of the twenty-first century. As a qualified Pilates instructor, I can confirm that time and time again, I have seen its magical ability to strengthen muscles and the core, increase flexibility, balance and coordination, decrease stress and improve overall health.

Pilates exercises are performed both on the mat and on specially designed equipment like the reformer, the Pilates chair, the Cadillac and so on. What makes this form of exercise so remarkable is that it engages both the body *and* the mind. The exercises are relatively safe, low impact and appropriate for anyone from the age of 10 to 100.

~ -W- *Pilates is one of the best forms of exercise for improving flexibility, boosting strength and seeing results you never thought you would see!*

*There are many Pilates-specific certifications to include BASI (Body Arts and Science International) Certified Pilates Instructor, among others.*

*Once you enjoy the feeling of suppleness that Pilates gives, you will keep coming back for more. But there are also Pilates group classes, as mentioned before, if you are the type of person who gains strength from fellow exercisers.*

## 14. Fitness for Older Adults

One of the most heart-warming trends I've seen in recent years is how keen older adults—especially those over sixty—are to exercise. Spurred on by their doctors but also encouraged by friends whose health has been revitalized by fitness, they are the veritable new kids on the block, sometimes out-pumping my younger clients on the training floor.

The notion that exercise is for the young is fast dissipating. Youth doesn't automatically suggest fitness anyway. We all have biological ages, yes, but we also have a metabolic age, which tells us how many calories our bodies burn at rest and is in itself a measure of fitness. Theoretically, the younger you are, the fitter you are, but there are clients of mine who have lower metabolic ages in their forties or fifties than those in their twenties or thirties. If you have access to a body composition machine, you will be able to find out yours too.

Getting older should *never* prevent you from exercising. In fact, it will delay ageing in the first place. And while we can't deny that our bodies have certain limitations as we get older, it doesn't necessarily mean that we understand those limits until we (safely) test them.

~ 🕐 -\\\- Building endurance, flexibility and strength is possible at any age. The only caveat is that progress should be made safely in small and gentle increments.

🏅 For a healthy, safe and quality workout, I always ask older adults to get the necessary medical checks done before committing to a routine. Finding a qualified instructor to guide them is also a must.

◎ You may need help in the beginning, and a good class or instructor may be able to craft workouts that suit you.

## 15. Exercise as Medicine

Another encouraging development over the past few years is that people now have a deeper understanding of the preventive and curative benefits of exercise. Yet, I sadly find that people are still far too comfortable with the idea of being dependent on pills even as doctors are increasingly prescribing mandatory exercise as an adjunct therapy for so many conditions that include heart disease, diabetes, depression, kidney stones, PCOS, anxiety and more. Even if you don't completely get off your medication, reducing your dependence on it means that your body is able to function better on its own. And who doesn't want that?

You don't even need to be on medication to feel better. We all know that exercise releases endorphins, the 'feel-good' hormones. Exercise is a proven stress-reliever and helps with your mental well-being—I've always found that a person who exercises regularly is less stressed than a person who doesn't. And I guarantee that after you work out, the problem that you're mulling over will not seem as big.

## 16. Fitness Influencers

Can we really leave social media out of any conversation any more? Fitness influencers are easy to find and follow. Most of them provide great fitness and nutrition tips and also open up their lives for the world to see the behind-the-scenes effort it takes to look as they do. They're especially great for motivation and inspiration, but always remember to follow any generic advice cautiously and do what works for you.

## 17. Gyms

Gym memberships are coming back to life, and they have their own special place in the fitness landscape. There are advantages gyms provide that are simply not enjoyed by individuals or home gyms that include equipment like Multi-Functional Trainers (MFTs) or Pilates equipment—that are more easily found in gyms—as well as studio classes, equipment, trainers and with them, a vibrant community.

*The Big Bang Fitness Menu* in no way suggests that these didn't exist before. Some, like exercise bikes, have been rediscovered. Others, like online classes, have taken off. But if you are looking to supplement the 10-minute workout stacks in this book with workout ideas, then you should have what you need here.

## Rules for negotiating fitness options in any world

It doesn't matter whether you're a beginner or giving experts a run for their money, there are some rules of fitness that apply to *everyone*, and there are no exceptions.

### Rule 1: Start at the Bottom

Few things affect your workout as deeply as your shoes and the first rule of fitness is getting the right support. Their job is to absorb the shocks imposed upon your body caused by running, jumping, or even walking. If done right, a well-chosen shoe can even better your workout. They don't have to be expensive, but they do have to suit the purpose of your workout. A few things to keep in mind:

1. **Decide what you want to use the shoe for.** Medicine is no longer the domain of the super specialists; sports shoes have also become a lot more targeted. *Runners and walkers* need to find shoes with good cushioning to absorb the shocks that are an inevitable part of movement. For *gym training,*

cushioning may interfere with the stability of your workout, so shoes designed for weight training are preferred. For *aerobic dance* or workouts like *Zumba,* there are dance sneakers. And the list goes on.

But if all of this is giving you a headache, a sturdy pair of *multipurpose* shoes is also a good way to start. You can use these to begin with, and then get more activity-specific footwear when the commitment to your workout deepens.

2. **Do your homework.** Shoe stores have trained and knowledgeable salespeople who are equipped to help you, and chances are that irrespective of the brand, they will tell you similar things. Of course, the job of a salesperson is to make a sale, so you may want to check out reviews online or ask your friends.

3. **Try not to buy shoes without trying them on first.** Yes, that online deal is tempting but find ways to try before you buy. There is absolutely no point in getting a good price if you're trying them on for the first time after you've bought them. Forcing an active lifestyle on shoes that fit but aren't *quite* right is one of the quickest ways to injure yourself.

When it is time to let go:

I was in the middle of instructing a class once when I saw something black whizz past the corner of my eye. I thought it was a mouse. Naturally, I started screaming because that is what you do when you see a mouse. The class came to a stop, and so did the black thing. It was not a mouse. It was a part of a sole of someone's shoe that had disengaged itself from the mothership and escaped to freedom.

If there ever was a time to let go of your old gym shoes, might I suggest it be before it lets go of you? It is time to take special care when:

1. *You wear them almost daily to work out or walk.* If your shoes absorb shock from high-impact movements on a regular basis, you will need to change them every six months. As your shoe ages, so does its ability to absorb shocks. Gym shoes, however, can last far longer than the pair you use to walk or run as they do not encounter as much impact.
2. *When you get too comfortable.* Comfort in the shoe does not translate to comfort in the body. No matter how comfortable they *feel*, they can only absorb shocks for so long.
3. *If you have new and inexplicable pain in your body.* Scaring a group class aside, disintegrating shoes can adversely affect your alignment, knees, feet, back and body.

## Rule 2: Know Thyself

Blindly following fitness influencers or your friends is a great way to keep doctors, painkillers and ice packs close. Believe in yourself but always *underestimate* yourself at the start of something unfamiliar. One way of starting slow is with the programme you choose. For example, if you're searching for a YouTube workout and you haven't exercised much or with a particular trainer, always type 'beginner', and even then be careful—one trainer's 'beginner' workout is sometimes another trainer's 'intermediate'. Only graduate to the next level if you have 'passed' the beginner level. The same goes for offline workouts, although many gyms or trainers put you through a fitness test or at the very least consult with you before they design your programme.

Knowing thyself also extends to the choice of weight. When is a weight too heavy? A weight is too heavy when your form goes out of sync. Or when you're compensating the load by lifting with body parts other than the ones you're supposed to be working out with. It could also be too light when you can do more repetitions than what is required of you. Selecting the right weight is a process of trial and error. If it's too light, you won't get strength gains, and if it's heavy, you risk injury. It has to be a little difficult but not *too* difficult.

## Rule 3: Stick to the Rules

Running is not bad for you if you have the right technique and if you don't have an underlying knee condition. Strength training can make you your leanest, toned self if you follow the rules. You can get fantastic results out of Pilates or yoga if you exercise with intent and pay attention to the form. You can get the best out of the 10-minute stacks in this book if you follow the instructions carefully. Most exercise programmes work if you stick to the rules because the rules have been designed keeping you in mind.

## Rule 4: Back-Up Your Fitness

A rainy day, an instructor on leave, the inability to leave the house and a shuttered gym are some of the reasons people tend not to show up for their workouts. If you are doing workouts other than those in this book, it doesn't hurt to have a back-up option or checking an online class or investing in some low-cost equipment. After checking with a fitness instructor or a medical professional, you could also enhance (where not mentioned) the workouts in this book using:

1. Resistance bands
2. Dumbbells/travel weights
3. Skipping rope
4. Aerobic step
5. Ankle weights

## Rule 5: You don't have to break your body to achieve results

Work out at your own pace. Setting time aside to work out is not always easy to do, and you have the right to enjoy it. You can exercise twice a day, but you shouldn't exercise for more than an hour at a time. Stay in your own lane and compete only against yourself.

The only clock you should be running on is yours.

# FITNESS STORY

### Katrina Kaif

As I mentioned in my Foreword, I first met Yasmin at a party where I couldn't help but admire her toned arms. We have worked together since then, and she has helped me achieve every professional fitness goal I have set out to attain. Yas would always work out along with me and be my driving motivation— if someone next to you is exercising so effortlessly, you have no excuse! In the spirit of the advice in this book, there are some things that I have learnt along the way in my fitness journey that I thought I could pass on to you:

First, focus on your *diet*. I don't mean literally going 'on' a diet but being conscious of your nutrition. It is an equally important, if not more important, component of fitness, and without monitoring it, exercise simply won't get you the body you want.

Second, be *open-minded* about different forms of exercise, and try new things if you are bored. I used to feel that I always had to do heavy workouts for fat loss and muscle tone. I used to call Pilates a 'recovery exercise', akin to physiotherapy, until I started it myself after a LOT of persuasion from Yas. That is when I realized that you could achieve great results with gentle forms of exercise, too. I would also change it up with yoga, gymnastics, aerial workouts, a mix of cardio routines, HIIT training, all of which have worked for me at different phases of my life.

Third, have a clear *agenda* about what you want from your training session. Do you want to break into a sweat and get your blood pumping? Or get the best workout for your arms, abs or thighs? By focusing on your goal while you exercise; you will get a better workout.

And lastly, *enjoy* your workouts. For me, exercise sets the tone and attitude for my day. Instead of dreading it, train your mind to enjoy this commune with your body. When you are feeling fit and strong, you feel better and more confident about yourself, and you will be more prepared to achieve what you need to.

6

# Fingers 0, Bodies 1

*End note from Yasmin*

I think most fitness instructors would agree with me when I say that the actual fitness *instruction* is half the job. The other half is *inspiring* people to get fit, to challenge their limits and to believe in themselves. That is why when I was thinking of how to conclude *The Perfect 10: 10-Minute Workouts You Can Do Anywhere,* I thought of putting inspirational quotes or deferring to the fitness greats that have been the reason I get up and go to work—Joseph Pilates, Jane Fonda or Pervez Mistry, closer to home. But I realized that that may not be universal enough; and that what inspires fitness trainers may not inspire celebrities, CEOs, housewives or students. I needed to find a message that united us.

There is no shortage of discussion around the reasons for getting fit—we hear enough about benefits like improving the quality of life to delaying ageing, eliminating or reducing dependence on medication, recovering from injury as well as boosting immunity, feelings of well-being, brain power, concentration and focus. But I'd like you to consider one more argument that I find applies to all of us, regardless of our age or health profile.

*Your body controls the worlds you have access to.* It will decide whether you can take that quick trip, put in that extra hour at work, juggle responsibilities, have meaningful relationships, catch up with friends, be an attentive parent and fully engage with life around you. A lack of stamina, tiredness, weakness, insufficient sleep, dehydration, poor concentration or improper nutrition will reduce your ability to participate, be present and give your best.

Think of your body as a vehicle. *It takes you where you want to go.* The more constrained you are by your body, the more limited your access, the narrower your world, the harder it will be to get to where you want and become who you want to be, even more so as you get older.

If you argue that desk jobs don't need physical movement, I say exercise is important for mental acuity. If you believe that functioning on less sleep is a badge of honour, I say you're setting yourself up for problems in the future. If you feel that your well-being is low on your list of priorities, I will argue that you won't be able to address those priorities *without* taking care of your well-being. Health is the key to unlocking any world you want. And fitness is the key to your health.

I often encounter people who seem inspired by what I do but for some reason seem intimidated by the thought of having to actually *do* it. They think it's beyond their reach or that the exercises can only be attempted by fitness professionals. They often don't see that behind a well-executed push-up or a flawless plank lie failures and frustration. *The Perfect 10: 10-Minute Workouts You Can Do Anywhere* has *not* been written to broadly inspire you to become fitter. The exercises have been broken down in stacks to *make* you work out for 10 minutes every day. Soon, you may even want to go beyond this book. That is when I know I have been truly successful.

Fitness starts with the basics and you build on these basics. And to do that, consistency is your best friend. Find those *10 minutes, preferably at the same time every day*, and see how a small habit transforms your body over time. Muscles are something to be *built*, strength is something to be *built*, endurance is something to be *built* and the process of building it is a little bit of effort day by day, week by week. And time is the tool you need to build with.

Over time, as you keep coming back to these pages and your fitness level improves, you will find yourself investing more time in your workouts. And you may find that an hour is better than 50, 30 or 10 minutes. But do you know what 10 minutes is definitely better than?

Zero.

*

# Acknowledgements

The Perfect 10: 10-Minute Workouts You Can Do Anywhere *could not have been possible without:*

- my two fathers in heaven for being my guardian angels and always looking out for me.
- my Mom, for always being the wind beneath my wings.
- my mother-in-law, for always encouraging and supporting me.
- my husband, Minhaz, for being my pillar of strength.
- my brother, Saif, for being my biggest cheerleader and honest critic.
- my nieces, Shaazia and Aaliyah, for loving me unconditionally.
- my sons, Zahaan and Amaan, for being patient and sharing me selflessly with others.
- my son Zahaan, who shot, edited and rolled out all the videos for this book.
- Gayatri Pahlajani, without whom this book would never have happened. Thank you for putting my thoughts into words so beautifully.
- my team—Nishreen, Urvi, Vaibhav, Vanshika and Pearl—for their patience, support and hard work.
- Luluaa Mathias, for my flawless make-up.
- Ashley Rebello, for my wardrobe and helping me be stylish.
- Ambereen Yusuf, for my hairstyles.
- Munna S, for capturing the exercises perfectly.

297

- Gurveen Chadha, and the team at Penguin Random House India for their support through this process.
- And also, a big thank you to all of you for patiently reading this book!

## *Ode to my Fathers*

My father, Fakhruddin Qureishi, was my first role model. From him, I learnt to live life on my own terms. He always taught my brother and I to follow our dreams. While he never stopped us from pursuing what we wanted to, he was very clear that we needed to do whatever we did with integrity. As a father, he indulged me but at the same time, he was a disciplinarian and never allowed me to go astray. He believed that you had to be honest first to yourself, then to others and then to the work you were doing. Because of him, I was able to pursue my dreams without feeling like I was being held back. I don't miss my father because I believe that he is with me every step of the way and I know he is that shining star in heaven constantly looking down over me. And is with me.

My father-in-law, Shabbir Karachiwala, is the reason I was able to pursue Pilates because when I first wanted to do the course—which required me to be in the US for three months—he encouraged me to do it. My kids were very little, and he and my mother-in-law moved into my house to look after them while I was away. And he would always, *always* be my biggest cheerleader. He also used to wonder how I never got tired running from pillar to post, doing a hundred things. 'When do you take a breath?' he'd ask. I said I didn't need to, because I had such good support, one of the reasons being him and my mother-in-law.

I am eternally grateful for these two shining stars in the sky looking down at me, and who are always with me. And I want to thank them from the bottom of my heart.